The
FOUNTAIN

25 Experts Reveal Their Secrets of Health and Longevity from the Fountain of Youth

JACK CHALLEM, EDITOR

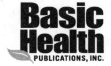

Basic Health
PUBLICATIONS, INC.

The information contained in this book is based upon the research and personal and professional experiences of the contributors. It is not intended as a substitute for consulting with your physician or other healthcare provider. Any attempt to diagnose and treat an illness should be done under the direction of a healthcare professional.

The publisher does not advocate the use of any particular healthcare protocol but believes the information in this book should be available to the public. The publisher and contributors are not responsible for any adverse effects or consequences resulting from the use of the suggestions, preparations, or procedures discussed in this book. Should the reader have any questions concerning the appropriateness of any procedures or preparation mentioned, the contributors and the publisher strongly suggest consulting a professional healthcare advisor.

Basic Health Publications, Inc.
28812 Top of the World Drive • Laguna Beach, CA 92651
949-715-7327 • www.basichealthpub.com

Library of Congress Cataloging-in-Publication Data
The fountain : 25 experts reveal their secrets of health and longevity from the fountain of youth / Jack Challem, Editor.
    p. cm.
  Includes bibliographical references and index.
  ISBN 978-1-59120-248-6
 1. Longevity. 2. Health. 3. Diet. 4. Aging—Prevention.

 RA776.75.F674   2009
 613.2—dc22

                                        2008053766

Editor: Diana Drew
Typesetting/Book design: Gary A. Rosenberg
Cover design: Mike Stromberg

Printed in the United States of America

10   9   8   7   6   5   4   3   2   1

Contents

To beautiful Rosa,
my beloved wife and best friend,
the creative spirit in our family,
whose idea and vision inspired this book.

—Norman Goldfind, Publisher

Introduction

In our own way, each and every one of us would like to find the fountain of youth. The reason is simple. We'd like to live as long as we can, erase our illnesses and age-related debilities, and enjoy as much as we can in life. In this book, we bring together twenty-five experts from medicine and natural health to relate their own personal experiences and to share their recommendations for achieving a long and healthy life.

Throughout history, people have sought a fountain of youth, and uncovering the secret to eternal youth has been a frequent theme in myths, legends, and even science fiction. Medieval herbs, such as lemon balm, and various concoctions created by alchemists were once thought to be elixirs of life. These nostrums evolved into the patent medicines of the nineteenth and early twentieth centuries and can still be seen in the panacealike claims proferred by modern pharmaceutical companies.

More than five hundred years ago, native residents of Puerto Rico told the Spanish explorer Juan Ponce de León of waters with remarkable healing and regenerative properties. In the process of searching for this mysterious fountain, Ponce de León discovered Florida. Is it any wonder that retirees still flock to Florida, or that people of all ages seek relief and respite in mineral springs?

In 1896, F. C. Havens published *The Possibility of Living 200 Years*, in which he summarized the recommendations of other authors and experts. Although the book seems quaint and antiquated by today's standards, Havens did touch on that proverbial grain of truth when he described the health hazards of "excessive oxidation or waste in the system." Sixty years later, Denham Harman, MD, PhD, developed the free radical theory, which holds that excessive oxidation leads to cell damage and aging. Harman's idea remains one of the key scientific explanations for why we grow old and become more susceptible to disease as we age. It is also the justification for taking *anti*oxidant supplements, such as vitamins C and E.

In 1933, the British author James Hilton published his novel *Lost Horizon* (which became a movie four years later), in which he described the earthly paradise of Shangri-La, where people lived so far beyond the average life span that they were considered practically immortal. Before writing *Lost Horizon*, Hilton had visited the Hunza Valley, located in northern Pakistan. The high mountain valleys and snow-capped peaks make for stunning scenery, and many books were published in the 1950s and 1960s on the Hunza people, extolling their exceptional health and longevity.

Sad to say, most of the reports about the diets and longevity of Hunza Valley residents turned out to be closer to fiction than fact. We now know that the Hunzas equated age with wisdom or wealth, so it was common for people to double their reported chronological age to 120. Rather than being vegetarians, the Hunzas cultivated and ate whatever they could scrape together—vegetables and fruits in the summer and early fall, meats and high-fat foods over the bitterly cold winter. Malnutrition was common, as it is in many other remote regions of Asia. In fact, a photograph and caption in the 1957 book, *Hunza: Lost Kingdom of the Himalayas*, describes the treatment of goiter, a disease brought on by a severe deficiency of iodine. So much for a healthy diet in an earthly paradise.

So let's leave legend and myth behind, and focus on the present and the future.

The contributors to *The Fountain* have based most of their recommendations on solid science and, to a great extent, on nutritional medicine and clinical practice. Most are physicians, researchers, nutritionists, and health experts of other types. Their recommendations focus primarily on the importance of nutrition and supplements, rather than on medical technologies or pharmaceuticals. The reason is very simple: We are biochemical creatures (at least in our physical makeup), and nutrients form the building blocks of all the body's biochemicals, including genes. That said, some of the contributors address the roles of healthy emotions, relationships, physical activity, and control of stress in promoting health and longevity. All these aspects of life figure in our lives and, directly or indirectly, influence our biochemistry.

There is no shortage of books on health and longevity, many of them filled with distracting footnotes. For *The Fountain*, we encouraged our contributors to write more from their hearts, instead of referencing hundreds of scientific studies. We asked them draw on their personal experiences in life (oftentimes informed by their reading of scientific journals and their experience in treating patients) and to make solid recommendations for readers.

You will, of course, encounter some differences of opinion within these pages. Some of our experts recommend vegetarian diets, while others suggest a modern version of the Paleolithic diet—essentially just fish, meats, vegetables, and fruits. Some emphasize natural foods, whereas others strongly recommend nutritional supplements. We wanted them to write about what has worked for them and their patients, allowing you to choose which ideas to try.

In the Afterword, I comment on many of the contributors' recommendations and distill key points into practical suggestions. Here you'll discover many paths, some closely related to each other, for maintaining your health and living a long, productive, and enjoyable life. We hope this book leads you to your own fountain of youth.

Jack Challem
Tucson, Arizona

My Habits and Tips for Longevity

Robert Abel, Jr., MD

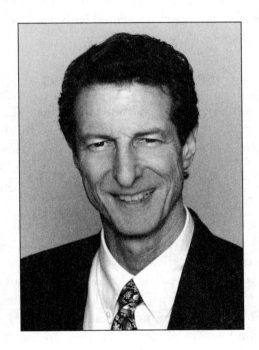

Robert Abel Jr. is a nutritionally oriented ophthalmologist and the author of *The Eye Care Revolution*. Address: Delaware Ophthalmology Consultants, 3501 Silverside Road, Wilmington, DE 19810. Tel: 302-479-3937. Website: www.eyeadvisory.com

Many years ago my mother derided doctors for their ignorance about nutrition. We discussed Carlton Fredericks and Adele Davis, and the primacy they accorded nutrition as the basis for wellness. That struck a resonant chord later on, when I took biochemistry in medical school and learned that essential nutrients build the body and that key deficiencies have long been known to cause physical diseases, such as scurvy, beriberi, or pellegra.

I also realized that operating on cataracts was treating a symptom and not treating a cause. Cataract surgery is the greatest cost to Medicare and yet we are reacting to the development of a situation that could very well have been prevented with a pair of sunglasses and a bit of insight dispensed by eye physicians.

INTUITIVE THINKING

The caduceus represents the symbol of medicine. The staff of Hermes with two snakes is attributed to Pythagorus. Its significance lies in the fact that one snake represents science and logical linear thinking, while the other snake represents art, intuition, and nonlinear thinking. This yin/yang duality applies to how we think about wellness and lifestyle choices.

The fountain is an excellent metaphor for personal health and our recommendations for lifestyle changes in others. Each of us involved in caregiving is constantly called on to treat a condition or give advice. As an ophthalmologist, I have found that the eye is not only the window to the soul but also the window to the body. The retinal receptors in the eye have the fastest metabolism in the body and are solely dependent on the liver for all their nutrition. In fact, the liver is the sentinel organ in the body, in addition to acting as the purification system and nutrient storage center. So you see that supporting eye health is akin to supporting total body health.

NEWBARS™

When I lecture, I often use the acronym NEWBARS™ as a way of identifying lifestyle habits with an eye toward prevention. This acronym stands for Nutrition, Exercise, Water, Breathing, Alternative options,

Relaxation, and Socialization. Each of these habits has multiple sub-components. Along with decisions about keeping a healthy pantry, supplementation is especially important for seniors, athletes, active people, and those with, or at risk of, common medical conditions.

With each of these NEWBARS™ items we must incorporate mind/body harmony. For instance, exercise, in order to become a habit, has to be done in a regular and thoughtful way. Stretching twice a day helps release tension in the body and supports the relaxation response. I personally spend time doing tai chi every morning after my shower, and during the course of the day I practice standing on one leg for balance or take two stairs at a time when walking between floors. An old Chinese proverb states that if one repeats an activity for one hundred days, it then becomes a habit. I have found this adage to hold true.

Nutrition

Many of the long-term prospective studies on longevity identify choices of foods, exercise, some form of dexterity and maintenance of total body health. Often this means avoidance of obesity (waist size 38 or greater and BMI >30) which leads to the metabolic syndrome. Healthy choices include vegetables, fish, grapes, seeds and berries, and a little bit of red wine. Reduce the five white thieves: white rice, white flour, white sugar, lard, and salt.

Exercise

Use it or lose it. Everybody knows that for cardiovascular health some form of exercise ideally is best to get your heart rate up to a level appropriate for your age. Walking, jogging, running, biking, and even yoga and tai chi are also healthy ways to reduce calories, achieve fitness and quiet the mind.

Water

The body is composed of more water than any other chemical. Six glasses of water a day is better than six glasses of any other liquid.

Soda, especially with artificial sweeteners, is not as healthy and brings a higher incidence of the metabolic syndrome in midlife. A filter can be placed on your kitchen sink or on your whole house to provide a healthy, tasty source of nutrition: Reverse osmosis will actually yield the cleanest, safest drinking water. Notice the fact you are more alert after drinking water for lunch than a soda or coffee: You may not need that extra caffeine stimulation during the day.

Breathing

Breathing is the key to quieting the mind and is an essential component in all martial arts and meditation techniques. We have to breathe anyway, so we might as well take a nice deep breath, let it out slowly, and enjoy it. It is not called *inspiration* for no reason! Doing this on a regular basis is excellent for people with high blood pressure, pulmonary disease, glaucoma, and many other chronic conditions.

Alternative Options

This refers to periodically reevaluating one's current medications and seeking alternative health solutions that are safer and might be equally effective. For example, consider arm massage for carpal tunnel syndrome, neck massage for unexplained headaches, magnesium for restless leg syndrome, saw palmetto for urinary frequency, or ginkgo for improving blood flow to the optic nerve into the brain. Of course, it is important to integrate all these modalities into an overall treatment plan monitored by your physician, but it is often the patient who must explore new solutions and bring this information to the physician. Medical doctors have been trained to diagnose and treat pathological conditions. People need to select options to encourage wellness and maintain health. Chinese and ayurvedic medicine is designed to address deficiencies using multiple herbs and change the composition based on changes in each patient. Traditional Western medicine treats all people with the same medication and may add additional medications to manage adverse reactions instead of eliminating the causative prescription. Seeking natural paths, herbal medicine doctors and acupuncturists may be effective in maintaining balanced health.

Relaxation and Socialization

Relaxation is self-explanatory. We all need to find ways to take time out and enjoy nature, walking, yoga and the company of others. Use dining as a way of creating memorable moments instead of merely as an outlet to deal with stress or depression. Giving to others is equally important: Try sharing your strengths to help others as a way to make yours a better community. Many people find volunteering tremendously relaxing and reinvigorating, as well as personally rewarding and satisfying.

Personal empowerment is the first goal in making a difference in one's life. Abraham Maslow outlined the hierarchy of needs, whereby each of us had to resolve basic insecurities and conflicts before achieving self-actualization. If you can reach the point where you recognize that you are no better than your fellow humans, that you know who you are and realize that only you stand in judgment of yourself, you have attained something very special and powerful. Accepting the inevitability of change is important to being a healer.

MY DAILY ACTIVITIES

I would like to share my daily activities and how I maintain a positive attitude and a healthy lifestyle. Every morning I get up at 5:00 a.m. without the need for an alarm clock; somehow my brain manages to do it by itself. I find that I can do my best thinking in the morning and have a small cup of coffee and a bowl of whole-grain cereal with nuts, berries, and pomegranate juice. I read the paper and plan my day. I eat very little dairy, primarily because of my lactase deficiency but also because of the questionable value of drinking the milk from another species and the association of milk protein and chronic sinusitis. I follow this up by drinking two glasses of water and taking 1,000 mg vitamin C, 1,000 mg MSM, 1,000 mg of quercetin, and 50 mg of B-complex vitamins (all of which are water-soluble).

After showering, I stretch on the floor and do qi gong. I then do the first form of yang-style tai chi and say my silent thoughts and prayers for the day.

With a small second breakfast having some fat in it, usually eggs, I have my morning multivitamin, 400 IU of E, 500 mg acetyl L-carnitine, 500 mg DHA, and 6 mg lutein. DHA, the algae-derived polyunsaturated fatty acid, facilitates the growth of the human brain. A deficiency in DHA contributes to many neurological, cardiac, and ocular conditions. Currently, I am taking my own formulation, Right for the Macula™, which contains 400 mg DHA and 6 mg of lutein twice daily. Recent articles have shown that lutein and zeaxanthin not only provide protection against UV radiation to the retina, but also to the skin. In fact, there is a fourfold protection rate from taking 6–10 mg of these two carotenoids on a daily basis.

At lunchtime, I have a salad as a way of getting valuable nutrition without increasing the sugar or fat load. I find that it keeps my head clear in the office in the afternoon and guarantees me one large portion of leafy-green vegetables. Throughout the day, I drink as much water as possible between patients.

Dinner usually consists of a sweet potato or a whole-grain starch, a green vegetable, and fish or organic nonbeef meat. I have avoided beef ever since the first mad cow scare in Washington state in 2004. Throughout the day, I take an additional 1,000–2,000 mg of vitamin C (depending on the season), and psyllium fiber capsules with my multiple glasses of water.

Nighttime is devoted to callbacks, essay writing, and eventually reading before going to bed by 10:00 p.m. I usually take a 500-mg magnesium capsule, which contributes to relaxation of both the muscles and the mind. Having exercised several times a week with and without a trainer, I stretch in the evenings and roll on a Nolla Rolla, which is a sculpted wooden dowel that relieves tension down the paraspinatus muscles in the back.

TIPS FOR GENERAL HEALTH

The following are some of my tips for overall health:

- Observe nature: Remember ancestral medicine.
- Make healthful dietary choices: Nourish your cell membranes.
- Select appropriate supplements.

- Drink filtered water.
- Practice rhythmic breathing.
- Monitor your digestion and maintain regular bowel habits.
- Protect your liver, reduce synthetic medications when possible.
- Strengthen your immunity with vitamins C and D, and quercetin.
- Age gracefully by thinking young and nourishing the child within.
- Be alert to allergies; they often serve as an early-warning sign of impending illness.
- Manage joint stiffness and dry eyes.
- Take antioxidants to combat cancer, coronaries, and cataracts.
- Sidestep trigger events: Reduce stress.
- Exercise regularly.
- Practice stretching and spinal alignment.
- Take inventory; check your body regularly and be aware of new symptoms.
- Manage your environment, both home and office.
- Look for healthful alternatives; select natural remedies whenever possible.
- Select health care providers who work collaboratively with you.
- Maintain an upbeat attitude: This becomes a self-fulfilling prophecy.

SUMMARY

One of my primary beliefs is that life is a divine comedy. All too often, people see neither the divinity nor the humor that pervades all our activities. We are on an individual quest and there is no formula that fits each one of us. We need to be attentive to our own deficiencies and idiosyncrasies. We all can't maintain the same exercise schedule, metabolism, or bowel pattern; therefore, we have to get used to designing our own goals and practicing our daily habits in a comfortable, affordable, and enjoyable fashion.

Perhaps the essence of the fountain is the fountain of energy, that unbounded flow of chi (life energy) that keeps us going and helps all those around us. We must accept challenges without fear, trust our intuition, and modify our own lifestyle. This will enrich our lives and make for a longer, more fulfilling experience.

2

Overcoming Hidden Food Allergies

James Braly, MD

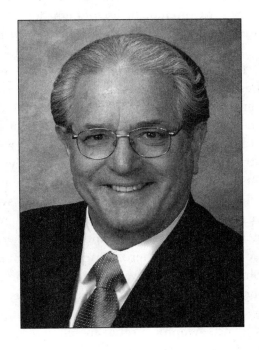

James Braly is one of the world's leading experts on food allergies, chemical sensitivities, and gluten intolerance. He is the author of *Dangerous Grains* and the classic *Dr. Braly's Food Allergy and Nutrition Revolution*. E-mail: info@lifestream-solutions.com. Website: www.lifestream-solutions.com

Like my mother before me, I suffered from frequent, disabling migraine headaches as a child, only to discover later that cow's milk—a favorite and perhaps addictive food of mine—was the culprit. As an adult, I often broke out in hives on my head, face, and shoulders when I went jogging. On one occasion, my airway completely closed off, leaving me unable to breathe for a terrifying minute or so. It turned out that wheat—another favorite and addictive food—was to blame. It should be of little surprise that when I opened my first medical practice a decade later, my primary focus and fascination were—and remain—clinical nutrition, addiction, and food allergies.

During the 1980s, we often made use of high-dose intravenous (IV) vitamin and mineral therapy to help clients through withdrawals coming off coffee, sweets, and other addictive foods. Most clients were able to resume therapy, free of symptoms, after one or two IV sessions. Years later, I was approached by the best-selling authors and educators—soon to be become close friends—Dr. David Miller and Merlene Miller. Having heard of my experience with IV nutritional therapy and addictions, they asked me to research and develop an intravenous nutrient formula and protocol that rapidly reversed withdrawal symptoms in recovering alcoholics and drug-dependent clients. (When addicted people become sober, many remain symptomatic in their abstinence for months, sometimes for years and even a lifetime. These abstinence symptoms, if severe and persistent enough, trigger relapse. What comes to mind here is a quote attributed to professional golfer John Daly, when he was struggling with one of his many attempts at sobriety from alcohol: "If this is sobriety, I'd rather be drunk.")

Chronic abstinence symptoms often include cravings for alcohol, drugs and/or sweets, anxiety, restlessness, depression, sleep problems, chronic fatigue, mental fogginess, inability to concentrate, irritability, and hypersensitivity to stress and noise, to name just a few. Three years after implementing our IV therapy, we find that over 80 percent of IV clients experience dramatic, rapid reduction in symptom severity, achieving a level of symptom relief not experienced in thirty days among those who choose not to have IV therapy.

We are now introducing both IV-oral nutrient therapy and food allergy testing and treatment in U.S. and UK recovery centers.

HIDDEN FOOD ALLERGIES

Independent studies have now confirmed what I discovered in my twenty years of clinical observations; namely, up to 80 percent of people with chronic illnesses and symptoms of any kind who respond poorly to conventional medical interventions are suffering from hidden (delayed-onset, IgG-mediated) food allergies. If left undiagnosed and untreated, these hidden food allergies can lead to premature death. For example, a severe form of wheat, rye, and barley sensitivity, called celiac disease, can knock about twenty years off your life, if left untreated.

A partial list of medical conditions in which hidden food allergies play a key role appears in the inset on pages 16–17.

Diagnosis and Treatment

Hidden food allergy (IgG-mediated, delayed-onset food sensitivity) is diagnosed by a simple blood test. The blood sample can now be obtained from an arm vein or a finger stick, using a self-administered home test kit. The blood samples are then sent to a licensed clinical lab for testing (a home test kit for celiac disease, now available in Europe, gives you results within five minutes—no doctor, no lab, no waiting time).

Beware. Not all labs are created equal. The best labs all use computerized ELISA (Enzyme-Linked ImmunoSorbent Assay) testing protocols and use only standardized foods when testing. With this in mind, here are my top three food allergy testing labs:

- **YorkTest Laboratories**—York, England; www.yorktest.com; customercare@yorktest.com (has a home test kit you can order online; uses finger stick; less expensive; good client support, 10–14-day turnaround)

- **Immuno Labs**—Fort Lauderdale, Florida; www.betterhealthusa. com (115-food test, more expensive, excellent client education and support, fast turnaround of test results)

- **MetaMetrix Labs**—Duluth, Georgia; www.metametrix.com (30- and 90-food test, midrange in price, nicely presented test results with informative guidebook)

Some Medical Conditions in Which Food Allergies Play a Part

When you identify and eliminate these foods, chronic symptoms improve or disappear in at least three out of every four patients who are blood-tested and treated.

One of my early patients was actor James Coburn, seeking relief from disabling rheumatoid arthritis. With a simple blood test, we discovered that he was allergic to several of his favorite foods, including wheat and tomatoes. One week after eliminating from his diet foods to which he was allergic, his arthritis disappeared. The actor appeared on the *Merv Griffin Show* to promote a recent movie he was starring in and ended up talking about food allergies and his arthritis. Merv subsequently followed our regimen and proceeded to lose thirty-five pounds—without restricting calories—and let the whole nation know about it. Moreover, over the next decade, thousands of patients visited our clinics for a wide variety of medical reasons, with the vast majority who had weight to lose losing weight and adding years to their lives simply by eliminating foods to which they were allergic and rotating nonallergic foods.

Arthritis

Attention deficit disorder, ADHD

Autism

Autoimmune diseases (insulin-dependent diabetes, thyroid disease, celiac disease)

Asthma

Bedwetting in children & adults

Canker sores (aphthous ulcers)

Celiac disease

Chronic conditions unresponsive to conventional medical therapies

Chronic fatigue syndrome (CFS)

Concentration & focusing problems

Depression—Adult

Depression—Children

Digestive disorders

Ear infections (middle-ear infections)

Eczema

Edema, fluid retention

Fibromyalgia

GERD (Gastroesophageal reflux disease)

Headaches

Heartburn

Insomnia	Osteoporosis unresponsive to therapy
Irritable bowel syndrome (IBS)	
Joint, muscle pain	Poor memory
Lactose intolerance	Psoriasis
Leaky gut	Sinusitis
Lung, breathing disorders	Skin disorders
Malnutrition, malabsorption	Sleep disorders
Mental fatigue	Weight loss
Migraine & cluster headaches	Yeast infections
Obesity, overweight	

Once your test results are back from the lab, I recommend the following guidelines:

- Eliminate all moderate to severe allergic foods (usually listed as +3 and higher on the test result report) for three months.

- Rotate all the nonallergic foods and foods that test equivocal (+1 or +2 every 4 days for at least 3 months). A four-day rotation of foods basically means you don't eat the same food or recipes containing that food more often than once every four days. As you will learn, this necessitates eating a wide variety of unprocessed foods.

- If you test positive for wheat, I strongly suggest that you follow up with a test for celiac disease. My top choice of labs screening for celiac disease is Prometheus Laboratories in San Diego; www.prometheuslabs.com.

Intravenous-Oral Nutrient Therapy for Addictions

Addiction is a disorder of brain chemistry and brain cell membranes. Long-term, symptom-free recovery requires nourishing and healing the brain. Nourishing the brain can be done with food, oral supplements, and IV therapy.

If you are in recovery or you frequently abuse alcohol (averaging more than one drink a day if you're a women and more than two drinks a day if you are a man) or addictive drugs (frequent use of marijuana, cocaine, or tranquilizers, and you score 60 or higher on the Abstinence Symptom Severity Scale), you could benefit greatly from IV-oral nutrient therapy.

In one study, I compared two groups of clients in recovery. One group of thirty-six clients received intravenous and oral nutritional therapy; the other group of sixteen received oral nutritional therapy only. The Abstinence Symptom Severity Scale was used to assess the severity of symptoms in each group before the start of nutritional therapy, daily for six days, and again at thirty days. Notice that the group receiving intravenous therapy had a greater reduction in the severity of abstinence symptoms in six days (69 percent reduction, averaging a total score of 36) than the group that received oral therapy alone had in thirty days (55 percent reduction and a total average score of 40). Diet and oral supplements were the same for both.

Our IV-oral nutrient therapy involves six to ten days of IV sessions, four hours each session. Just before each session, oral nutrients are given (certain nutrients such as fish oil and NADH are not available in the United States for IV infusion, while others like glutamine are unstable in solution). We are now using a combination of twenty-five different IV nutrients and nutrient derivatives, along with five to ten oral supplements for the treatment of addiction to alcohol, cocaine, methamphetamine, heroin, marijuana, and other illegal drugs, as well as some addictive prescription drugs. (*Note:* To date, this therapy has not been effective in treating addiction to benzodiazepines, such as Xanax, Klonopin, Ativan, and Valium. In addition, it does not appear to be helpful with clients being treated primarily for eating disorders.) For an updated list of U.S. and UK centers and clinics where this therapy is now available, visit www.lifestream-solutions.com.

3

Beyond Nutrition—A Holistic Approach to Longevity

Hyla Cass, MD

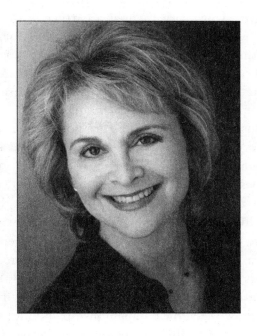

Hyla Cass is one of the country's foremost authors and speakers in the field of integrative medicine and psychiatry. She combines the best of leading-edge natural medicine with modern science in her clinical practice, writings, lectures, and nationwide media appearances. She is a former assistant clinical professor at UCLA School of Medicine and the author of several groundbreaking books, including *Supplement Your Prescription, Natural Highs,* and *8 Weeks to Vibrant Health.* Address: Pacific Palisades, CA 90272. Tel: 310-459-9866. E-mail: hyla@drcassmd.com. Website: www. drcass.com was asked to reveal my approach to health and longevity or, at least, to delaying the usual pitfalls of aging as long as possible. While death is inevitable, the goal here is to have a joyous, fulfilling, and healthy life for as many years as possible along the way. I'll share what has worked for me, my friends, my colleagues, my readers, and my patients.

A board-certified psychiatrist and practitioner of integrative medicine, I long ago abandoned the mainstream approach of the "physician as the all-knowing expert, a prescription, for every ailment, and the ten- to twenty-minute office visit." Instead, I spend an hour or two with patients, work with them as a partner in their health, look for root causes rather than treating symptoms, and, for the most part, depend on natural treatments, including lifestyle modifications and supplements. I prescribe medications where appropriate and only as a last resort. The "prescriptions" that I give out require more participation than simply taking a daily pill. Simply put, the key to preserving our health is participation. There are no shortcuts.

Of course, even doing our best in these areas, we all succumb to the inevitable at some point. The idea is to live every day fully, since it may be our last. Paradoxically, when taken to heart, this awareness can make life a true joy. We've seen people told that they had several months to live find great meaning in every aspect of the time remaining, and stuffing lifetimes of quality experience into those hours and days. *The Bucket List*, a film with Jack Nicholson and Morgan Freeman, is a perfect example of the turnaround that a "known" death sentence can inspire. In these two old men, diagnosed with advanced cancer, we see how companionship and mutual encouragement can be wonderfully life-enhancing, even (or particularly) in the face of death.

So how do we stay as youthful as we can? There are no magic pills, specific hormones, or special diets that provide the "answer." Youthfulness and longevity derive from a mysterious combination of factors, only some of which we can know or control. My own philosophy is that death can happen at any time, so don't take anything for granted—your health, your relationships, and the beauty that surrounds us all if we only take the time to look.

Questions abound, but I also have a few answers, guidelines to healthy living that will help you make the best of the body and life that you have.

Here is a short checklist of Life Enhancers and Life Extenders that I have found to be useful:

- A positive attitude, including psychological well-being and resiliency in the face of life's stresses

- Good and fulfilling relationships

- A healthy lifestyle, including good diet, appropriate supplements, and regular exercise

- Hormonal supplementation to compensate for naturally waning hormone levels as we age

ATTITUDE

Research shows that attitude has a powerful effect on the immune system. A positive attitude goes a long way toward keeping us young, vital, and healthy, just as a pessimistic, negative attitude can cause premature aging. Happiness in not happenstance: It is cultivated. We've seen people living in miserable circumstances radiating joy, while many with "perfect" lives are miserable. Two books that I recommend on how to create your own happiness are *What Happy People Know* by Dan Baker, and *Happy for No Reason: 7 Steps to Being Happy from the Inside Out* by Marci Shimoff.

RELATIONSHIPS

Spend quality time with others, in healthy relationships. Be supportive and loving toward your friends and family. In fact, helping others is a great remedy for anxiety and depression. Volunteer at a hospital or homeless shelter; there is no greater reward than what we receive from giving to others. And don't forget hugs—natural, safe, free, and mutually beneficial! It's known that married men live longer than single ones, and it is likely that all the love and support keeps them going.

STRESS MANAGEMENT

Stress is inevitable. It's not so much what the stresses are, but how we handle them that is most important. As Mark Twain said, "I have had many troubles on my life, most of which never happened." Allowing our built-in stress response—the flight or flight mechanism—to take over, not only interferes with our productivity, efficiency, and joy, but can negatively impact every system of our body—blood pressure, digestion, cholesterol levels, and even our immunity to infection. All this robs us of our energy, and our precious years.

Beyond the Stress Response

There are some simple stress reduction techniques, such as deep breathing, progressive muscle relaxation, and meditation that help reverse the innate stress response. To deal with chronic stress and anxiety, which is often related to some traumatic event in the past, other methods help to determine the root cause of your anxiety and clear it for good.

- Deep, relaxed breathing is an excellent anxiety and stress reducer, and overall tension reliever. Try it. You won't be able to both breathe deeply and feel anxious or tense at the same time! Regular meditation practice takes this a step further. Try ten minutes twice a day. There are many excellent books and courses on meditation— or simply sit quietly and focus on your breath. Your mind and body will naturally settle into a quiet, restorative state.

- Emotional clearing. There are a variety of specific brief and simple techniques that help you effectively deal with chronic feelings of stress and anxiety based on long-forgotten emotional issues, or ones that you either don't care to deal with or don't think are that important. One of my favorite methods is Gary Craig's EFT (www.emofree.com). Although it is best done initially with a therapist, once you have a good start, you can continue on your own. A powerful tool, EFT combines positive imagery and specific pressure points on the body to release negative thoughts and feelings. Another outstanding technique, called EMDR (Eye Movement Desensitization and Reprocessing; www.EMDR.org), uses rapid eye movements to help synchronize the two sides of your brain. Both methods, and others, allow negative feelings of fear, pain, and anger to be released, putting you back in your emotional driver's seat. EMDR is especially effective in helping people overcome post-traumatic stress disorder (PSTD).

- Positive thinking. You can also use positive thinking to reprogram your mind. Add some visualization, picturing and sensing how you would like your life to be. Research has shown this to be a very powerful way to create change in yourself and the world around you. Along with a positive attitude goes a spiritual connection, being in the present and connected to a larger purpose. Life must have meaning, connection to the Universe outside ourselves, whatever one's concept of the Divine is. This may include regular meditation, prayer, or simply being present to the wonders of nature.

LIFESTYLE

Be careful not to indulge in alcohol, drugs, or overeating. Beyond their effects on blood sugar and mood, drugs and alcohol also have toxic effects on the brain, liver, and other systems of the body. Don't substitute food for drugs, either: Excessive sugar and simple carbohydrates (sugar, white flour, and more) will only make matters worse. They play havoc with your blood sugar levels, upset your mood, and drain your energy. They also make you fat, and prone to heart disease, diabetes, and a myriad of other chronic diseases.

Diet

Have regular meals of fresh, organic food. This includes lots of fruits and vegetables, and a moderate amount of protein (fish, chicken, lean meat). The Mediterranean diet appears to be one of the healthiest. Ideally, you should eat at regular intervals, don't skip meals, have a substantial breakfast, a good-sized lunch, and a smaller dinner, and not too close to bedtime. This eating pattern helps avoid large fluctuations in blood sugar levels, which are hard on the body and cause premature aging.

NUTRITIONAL SUPPLEMENTS

With age, our bodies are less resilient and forgiving. When we were younger, we were better able to compensate for deficiencies. Now, we must be more diligent in our supplementation. With stress, too, we need to replenish those nutrients lost in the stress response, which uses up many of the nutrients that we need to be our best, both emotionally and physically.

You can cover your bases by taking a high-potency multivitamin and multimineral combination that includes B-complex vitamins; vitamins C, D, and E; calcium, magnesium, potassium, zinc, chromium, and manganese; plus trace elements, such as boron, vanadium, and molybdenum.

Essential fatty acids in the form of fish, fish oil, and flax oil are also important for brain health, hormone function, and even for soft, smooth skin.

You'll also need to pay special attention to antioxidants.

Antioxidants

A major contributor to aging are the reactive oxidative species (ROS), also known as free radicals. They are created both as by-products of normal metabolism and by the toxins that we ingest from our environment. Free radicals cause cellular damage, cell death, and, ultimately, body death. The solution is taking large quantities of neutralizing antioxidants, in the form of both food (fruits and vegetables) and supplements. Antioxidants are potent anti-inflammatories, too, as well as immune system boosters, battling infection and even potential cancers.

At this point, the American Cancer Society has joined the bandwagon of those recommending increased consumption of fruits and vegetables for cancer prevention. The most commonly recognized antioxidants are vitamins C and E, selenium, alpha-lipoic acid, and plant extracts, such as ginkgo, green tea, and ginseng. You need the whole array: They all work together like instruments in an orchestra, each with its own role in the process, to quench the dangerous free radicals. So a single antioxidant, even in large quantity, won't do it, or can even act as a dangerous pro-oxidant.

SLEEP

Be sure to get enough sleep, since sleep deprivation can undermine overall health—and even cause weight gain. If you have trouble falling asleep, and/or staying asleep, take 5-hydroxytryptophan (5-HTP), kava, or valerian, combined with some deep breathing. You can add some specific muscle relaxation exercises as well: In sequence, clench each muscle of your body for ten seconds as you inhale, then release as you exhale to the count of fifteen. Again, avoid using prescription sleeping medications. They can be addictive, and lead to rebound insomnia when you try to quit.

MINIMIZE MEDICATIONS

Half of the U.S. population is taking at least one prescription drug, and in the over-sixty-five age group, half take three or more. These have serious side effects, including nutrient depletion in an already nutrient-depleted population. Before rushing to take prescription medications, with side effects including possible addiction, try one of the many safe, effective natural remedies.

EXERCISE

Use it or lose it. We were meant to move and without regular movement, we deteriorate. Don't you feel better when you're exercising regularly? At the age of eighty-plus, my mother created a weekly aerobics class in her condo complex and invited her octagenarian friends to join her. It's been going on now for several years, and they are all the better for it. Exercise increases circulation, boosts oxygenation of our cells including brain cells, enhances neurotransmitter production, helps us maintain our weight, and offers countless additional benefits.

HYDRATION

It's important to drink the obligatory eight glasses of pure water daily, to provide the substrate for our body chemistry. Often older people are poorly hydrated, and this can show up as impaired brain function. Just add water and see what happens!

NUTRITION AND THE MIND

As a psychiatrist by training, I focus a great deal on the mind. Mental capacity and mood are closely related to hormone levels, and respond well to hormone therapy. I also prescribe supplements based on specific deficiencies. For example, levels of vitamin B_{12} decrease with age, due to difficulty in absorption, causing such symptoms as depression and mental fog. An injection or lozenge of vitamin B_{12} will often clear up the problem.

For depression I will also include amino acids such as 5 HTP and SAMe, plus an array of B vitamins and fish oil. For anxiety, I will add in theanine, kava, valerian, and GABA. Memory is a big issue in aging, and fortunately, we can save our brains! Besides exercising our brains with quizzes, crossword puzzles, social interaction, physical exercise is a known mental health enhancer. Antioxidants are essential for keeping our brains young; then we just need to add some other specific nutrients. Here are some of the supplements that I recommend to preserve and protect our brain: phosphatidyl choline, phosphatidyl serine, acetyl-l-carnitine, and ginkgo biloba.

HORMONES

Many of our body processes are regulated by hormones—chemicals released in minute amounts from specific glands and carried through the bloodstream to target areas where they do their job. The pituitary, the master gland found in the brain, just above and behind the eyes, produces specific "stimulating" hormones that activate the thyroid, adrenals, testes, and ovaries to produce such hormones as thyroid hormone, cortisol, DHEA, testosterone, estrogen, and progesterone.

As we age, these hormones go south, and so do we. In my practice, I recommend testing hormone levels, then restoring levels to those closer to youthful ones. What about an increased incidence of cancer after taking female hormones? The Women's Health Initiative Study, on which this fear is based, was using synthetic Premarin and Provera, rather than the bio-identical hormones that integrative physicians pre-scribe. We still monitor for any abnormal responses, but the risks are not as great as with the synthetic hormones, and the benefits, many. Men likewise may need hormone help, and there are some excellent sources of information on this as well.

In conclusion, for mental and spiritual health, you can combine prayer, meditation, emotional clearing, and breathing techniques. This, plus a healthy combination of good nutrition, including the right supplements (including hormones), exercise, water, and adequate sleep will provide an excellent buffer against aging, while restoring mind, body, and spirit. For a life worth living well, the time and atten-tion required for this pays off enormously.

4

My Personal and Professional Journey in Nutrition

Jack Challem

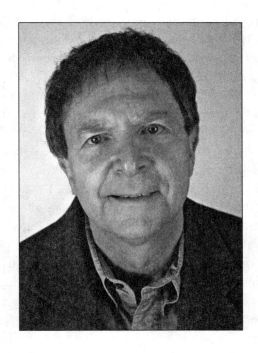

Jack Challem, known as The Nutrition Reporter™, is the author of more than twenty books on nutrition and health, including *Stop Prediabetes Now, The Food-Mood Solution,* and *The Inflammation Syndrome.* He is also a personal nutrition coach and provides nutritional consultations in person or on the telephone. Address: P.O. Box 30246, Tucson, AZ 85751. E-mail: jack@thenutritionreporter.com. Website: www.nutrition reporter.com.

am a best-selling author of nutrition and health books and I write for many different magazines. I also lecture consumer and medical groups on nutrition topics, and I coach people one-on-one to help them develop better eating habits. But most of what I do in this field and the nutrition recommendations I make are based on what I have learned from other people.

Many events and individuals have shaped my perspectives on nutrition and health. The first and perhaps most pivotal event was the death of my older brother. When I was fifteen years old, I saw him waste away from cancer, living in great pain for nine months. Much of his pain was the consequence of medical treatments. The lasting effect of that experience on me has been the firm belief that no one should ever die that way. Looking back, my brother's death fundamentally influenced much of my personal and professional journey in life.

By that time I was also interested in becoming a writer. A high school English teacher, Harold Miller, taught me to think critically—that is, not to take anything at face value—and he also helped sharpen my writing skills. Several years later, in college, Dr. Dewitt Garrett, a biology professor, made an offhand remark about "suppressed treatments" for heart disease and cancer. After class, I asked for more information about those treatments, and we talked about nutrition and vitamins. Within a couple of weeks, I started taking vitamin C and E supplements, and I had a very dramatic response to the vitamins. I had recently been diagnosed with a pilonidal cyst—a particular type of chronic, draining cyst or abscess. One week after starting the vitamins, the cyst burst, completely drained, and healed. That was around forty years ago. Most people who have a pilonidal cyst suffer with it throughout their life. Needless to say, I became convinced about the benefits of nutritional therapies.

THE EXPERTS I'VE LEARNED FROM

After graduating from college, I was lucky enough to start writing for some of the health magazines and, perhaps more importantly, meeting and becoming friends with the physicians who pioneered nutritional therapies. They included Evan Shute, MD, and his brother Wilfrid Shute, MD, the first doctors to use vitamin E to treat coronary heart disease. I got to know Abram Hoffer, MD, PhD, who was the first doctor to use high doses of vitamins B$_3$ and C to treat schizophrenic patients—and to enable them to experience the same reality that you and I see. Dr. Hoffer, still sharp at age ninety-one, has a rare appreciation of medical history and incredible clarity in thought, and I have learned much from him over the years. Carl Pfeiffer, MD, and Hugh Riordan, MD, were pioneers as well, and Dr. Riordan was eclectic in his thinking and a particularly strong influence. I am also indebted to Ron Hunninghake, MD, who has become a close friend and the best person for me to brainstorm with on nutrition issues.

I also learned a great deal from researchers, including Denham Harman, MD, PhD, who developed the free-radical theory of aging and disease; Lester Packer, PhD, who explained a great deal about antioxidant biochemistry to me; Bruce Ames, PhD, who did the same in terms of energy production in mitochondria; and Loren Cordain, PhD, who helped me make sense of the Paleolithic diet and many other important aspects of nutrition, such as acid-alkaline balance. I met Nobel laureate Linus Pauling, PhD, and talked with him several times on the telephone. Dr. Pauling was a true genius and, like Dr. Hoffer, he had exceptional clarity in thought (not surprisingly, they frequently collaborated). They and many others over the years have been my teachers—not in classes, mind you, but in explaining everything from the minutiae of nutritional biochemistry to the bigger real-life implications of orthomolecular medicine.

I am also very self-directed. I thrive on learning, and am an avid reader of newspapers, magazines, and medical and scientific journals. Years ago, I learned the advantage of living near a medical library, where I could retrieve full-text journal articles—after all, not everything is available for free on the Internet. This is part of the story of how I became interested in natural therapies and wellness. But there is another important aspect of my journey to relate before I discuss my recommendations for a healthy, fully functional life.

MY ENCOUNTER WITH PREDIABETES

In 1997, Dr. Riordan invited me to get a comprehensive nutritional workup at the center he founded in Wichita, Kansas. It's known formally as the Center for the Improvement of Human Functioning International, although most people refer to it as the Bright Spot for Health. It is the largest nonprofit nutritional medicine center in the United States and very likely in the entire world.

By that time, I was knowledgeable about, and also taking, many vitamin and mineral supplements. However, I was giving mostly lip service to a healthy diet, and my poor eating habits were catching up to me: At age forty-seven, I was about twenty pounds over my ideal weight, and my fasting blood sugar of 111 mg/dl indicated prediabetes (an early stage of type 2 diabetes). I immediately added some new supplements, emphasizing those that improve insulin function and blood sugar.

However, it took me a couple of years to make substantial dietary changes. In 1999, I was going through some personal changes in my life. I loved eating pasta, but one day it simply didn't taste as good anymore. So I stopped eating pasta, which is mostly starch and empty calories, and instead began eating more salads and baked chicken. Without intending to lose weight, I lost twenty pounds in three months—and it has stayed off in all the years since because I have maintained healthier eating habits. A few months later, blood tests showed my fasting glucose to be 87 mg/dl, a decrease of twenty-four points.

Déjà vu. I was convinced about the benefits of good eating habits.

Along my path in life, I have also learned that maintaining health is not a static process. It's dynamic and can change—should change—as we get older, switch jobs, or modify our lifestyle habits. At fifty-eight, my fasting blood sugar is now about 79 mg/dl, my fasting insulin is about 5 mcIU/ml, and my HbA1c is 4.9 percent. My numbers are *better than normal*, and the same is true with almost all my other blood-test numbers. Most people's numbers get worse with age; mine keep getting better. I have accomplished all of this without taking any drugs. This is the power of eating right and taking supplements.

One of the most important lessons I have learned is that supplements can greatly improve health—they do have preventive and therapeutic benefits—and healthy eating habits greatly magnify those benefits. Good food and good supplements are synergistic. Stress management is important, and so is physical activity—I began cycling several years ago, and the regular physical activity led to significant decreases in my cholesterol and triglycerides. It is also important to stimulate the mind by attending or participating in cultural activities, such as those involving art and music. Doing so actually prompts the brain to make new brain cells and, of course, most of us want to keep our smarts as we get older. It is also fundamentally important to maintain balance in one's life, such as to balance job-related pressures and deadlines with downtime, reading time, and recreational travel time.

As we age, we have to redouble our efforts to stay in good health. With aging, our genes suffer increasing damage, which negatively affects the biological program that guides our health life. As we get older, our biochemistry becomes less efficient and, unless we make a concerted effort, our bodies' levels of nutrients decline. It helps to "load" our biochemical pathways with nutrients so, from a biological standpoint, we function more like younger than older organisms.

FOUR DIETARY RECOMMENDATIONS

Sometimes people ask me why nutrition is so important. The answer is relatively simple: Our entire biochemistry, including the synthesis, repair, and regulation of our genes, depends on nutrients. Here's a useful analogy: Think of building a house with either shoddy or quality materials. If you use cheap construction materials, the house will not be structurally sound. Similarly, if you opt for poor-quality nutrition, your body will not be structurally sound. Conversely, if you build a house with sturdy components, it will resist damage from earthquakes and hurricanes. Likewise, if you eat healthy foods, you will better weather life's inevitable stresses.

So, what do I recommend in terms of healthy foods? It has taken me about thirty years of nutrition writing to distill almost everything into four simple recommendations.

Eat Nutrient-Dense Foods

These are foods that provide the greatest amount of high-quality nutrition in every bite or calorie. Two broad food groups meet this criterion. One is quality protein—in my mind, fish, chicken, turkey, eggs, and lean meats (preferably grass-fed, not corn-fed). The other food group consists of high-fiber (nonstarchy) vegetables and fruits. These include salads, broccoli, cauliflower, raspberries, blueberries, cherries, kiwi, and most other vegetables and fruits.

Meanwhile, avoid or limit your intake of low-nutrient-density foods, which include most starchy grain-based foods, including breads, cereals, bagels, muffins, and pastas; as well as sugary foods, such as candies and most types of energy bars. Potatoes, rice, and bananas are high in sugarlike starches, and people with prediabetes or weight issues should strictly limit their consumption of sugarlike starches. Although many people tout the health benefits of whole grains, they are nutritionally weak compared with vegetables.

Eat Fresh Foods

The healthiest foods are almost always fresh foods, and the unhealthiest foods are almost always packaged foods. Fresh foods are higher in nutrients because they have not undergone industrial processing and refining. By contrast, packaged foods have usually been processed, refined, or tampered with in some way. Packaged foods come in boxes, cans, jars, bottles, tubs, and bags. Nearly all packaged foods have added salt, sugars, junk oils, or trans fats—or all of them. There are a few exceptions that are healthy, such as olive oil and frozen vegetables and fruits, as long as nothing else has been added to them.

Fresh foods mean you have to prepare your meals from scratch. That will take a little extra time, but you can find that time (perhaps by checking e-mail less each day). When someone complains that cooking from scratch takes too much time, I tell him that he can either make the time to cook today or make the time to be sick and disabled in a few years.

Eat Foods That Look Like They Did in Nature

Excuse me if this sounds a little folksy, but I believe that foods should have some resemblance to what they looked like in nature. A piece of chicken should look like it was once part of an animal, and a piece of fish should look like it came from a fish. Most fresh foods do look something like they did in nature. Chicken nuggets don't look like anything that was grown or raised, and neither does fish and chips (French fries).

Hydrate Yourself—Mostly with Water

Our bodies consist mostly of water, and aging is often characterized by a shrinking of cells other than fat cells. The oxygen and hydrogen atoms that form water are needed for myriad biochemical reactions in the body, and many physicians have told me that the have seen improvements in their patients after doing nothing other than drinking more water. Although many people have complained about the huge amount of waste created by disposable plastic bottles, it is heartening to see many people drinking water instead of soft drinks. Other healthy beverages include sparkling mineral water, green and black teas, herbal teas, organic coffee, green (vegetable) drinks, and coconut water.

DECIDING WHICH SUPPLEMENTS TO TAKE

The scientific and medical evidence in support of using high-dose vitamins, vitaminlike nutrients, and minerals is overwhelming. Anyone who argues otherwise simply is not reading the scientific and medical literature. Nutrients have normal roles in our biochemistry, and I usually recommend a nutritional approach before suggesting herbs, homeopathic remedies, or other natural therapies.

Unfortunately, many people feel overwhelmed by the vast numbers of supplement companies and supplements on the market. They'll take one product because they've read that it will strengthen the heart, and they'll take another because they've heard that it will ease aches and pains. I once received a letter from an eighty-five-year-old reader who explained that he ate well, walked several miles each day, and also included a long list of the supplements he was taking. He asked me what to change to live a long and healthy life. I wrote him that, at age eighty-five, he shouldn't change a thing!

To keep supplements simple, I recommend that people begin with a high-potency multivitamin. It is essential to shore up your basic nutrition before buying and taking more arcane and highly hyped supplements. Look for a multivitamin containing 20–50 mg of vitamin B_1, and with that dose, the amounts of the other ingredients tend to fall in line. I also recommend that people take a separate multimineral supplement. Minerals are bulky, and there are manufacturing limitations governing the size of tablets and capsules (as well as limits to what most people can swallow). Because of the bulk of minerals, most supplements that combine a multivitamin and multimineral tend to shortchange people on minerals. These multis provide nutritional insurance against lapses in eating habits and many genetic and biochemical weaknesses.

After starting multivitamin and multimineral supplements, you can then choose from any number of individual supplements with very specific health benefits. It pays to read and learn about these supplements so you don't spend money on products you don't need. Consider the following:

- Vitaminlike coenzyme Q_{10}, which strengthens the heart and protects against breast cancer
- Lutein, which improves visual acuity
- Lycopene (good for the prostate)
- Omega-3 fish oils, which are anti-inflammatory and help regulate heart rhythm
- Gamma-linolenic acid (also anti-inflammatory)
- N-acetylcysteine, an antioxidant that offers the very best protection against cold and flu symptoms
- Silymarin, an herbal extract that significantly regulates blood sugar levels
- Resveratrol, a plant extract that appears to have age-slowing benefits

As far as I can tell, each of us has one life on this earth and one opportunity to live the best and healthiest life we can. Eating health-promoting foods and taking supplements are two important steps toward living a long, fully functional, and enjoyable life. Don't treat nutrition as a rigid doctrine—that's the problem with old-school dietitians and physicians who think in terms of 1950s Betty Crocker nutrition. Intead, keep up with the latest findings—a new discovery tomorrow could change much of what you currently know and take for granted. Above all else, remember that good nutrition should be part of a balanced approach to life in general.

5

A Diet Solution Based on Our Evolutionary Ancestry

Loren Cordain, PhD

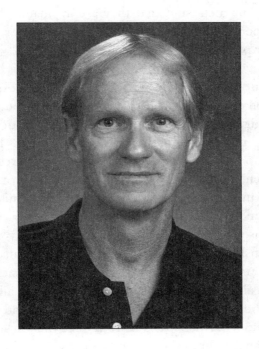

Loren Cordain is a professor in the Department of Health and Exercise Science at Colorado State University, Fort Collins, CO 80523. He has written three books, *The Paleo Diet, The Paleo Diet for Athletes,* and *The Dietary Cure for Acne.* Tel: 970-491-7436. Fax: 970-491-0445. E-mail: lcordain@cahs.colostate.edu. Website: www.thepaleodiet.com

DIETARY CHAOS

Two-thirds of American men and women over the age of twenty-five are overweight. And it's killing us. The leading cause of death in the United States—responsible for 41 percent of all fatalities—is heart and blood vessel disease. Fifty million Americans have high blood pressure, 40 million have high cholesterol levels, and 16 million have type 2 diabetes.

That's the bad news. The good news is that the scientific community is in almost unanimous agreement that these diseases and disorders are related to our diets, and that they are avoidable. Unfortunately, nutritional experts are in complete disagreement over which type of diet is best for preventing and treating disease.

The U.S. government's position on healthy eating is exemplified by the Department of Agriculture's My Pyramid, which exhorts us to eat between six and eleven servings of cereal grains daily and two to three servings of dairy foods, and to limit our consumption of fats and sweets. Other nutritional authorities, such as Dr. Dean Ornish, encourage us to lower dietary fat to less than 10 percent of calories and to eat plenty of whole grains and legumes. Noted alternative health physician Dr. Andrew Weil agrees with Ornish's advice on whole grains and legumes but takes issue with his fat recommendation, saying it is too low and deficient in omega-3 fatty acids (the kind found in fatty fish like salmon). Still other nutrition gurus, such as Dr. Neal Barnard, president of the private nonprofit Physicians Committee for Responsible Medicine, caution us to eliminate all animal products from our diets, including meat, eggs, dairy, and fish. In stark contrast, Dr. Robert Atkins tells us to reduce our carbohydrate content to less than 100 grams a day and to eat all the fatty, salty meats and cheeses we desire.

Is there any way to make sense of all this? I'm sure you've struggled with the same question I asked myself many years ago: What is the optimal diet for improving my health, losing weight, and reducing my risk of chronic illness?

HORSE SENSE FOR LIONS

Zookeepers learned long ago that in order for a wild animal not just to exist, but to thrive, be healthy, and reproduce in captivity, it was necessary to replicate as closely as possible the animal's natural habitat in the zoo. That included replicating the animal's diet in the wild. Exotic lemurs from Madagascar or rare monkeys from the Brazilian rain forest could be kept alive in captivity when fed standard monkey chow, but they did not do well. They were prone to infections, developed chronic diseases, and rarely, if ever, reproduced. However, when these animals were given a diet of insects, grubs, worms, and fresh plants—foods they ate in their natural habitats—they became more active and healthy and began to produce offspring. Why?

Feeding a beefsteak to a horse makes about as much sense as feeding hay to a lion. Horses, like lions, are evolutionary specialists. In response to their particular ecological niche, horses have evolved a specific physiology (such as flat, grinding teeth and a large gut) to handle a fibrous vegetarian diet of grasses and shrubs. By contrast, lions are carnivores, and evolution has equipped these cats with the tools (like fangs and claws and a smaller gut) to handle a concentrated diet of meat, marrow, bones, and organs. The genetic makeup of each of these animals has been shaped by the foods found in their environmental niches. When an animal is fed foods with which it has little or no evolutionary experience (beefsteak for a horse, hay for a lion), dissonance occurs between the newly introduced foods and the animal's genetic profile. If the animal continues to eat unfamiliar foods, this dissonance will ultimately cause illness, disease, and dysfunction.

STONE AGERS LIVING IN THE SPACE AGE

Humans are no different from horses or lions in terms of the specific ecological niche we occupy. The foods found in the diets of our hunter-gatherer ancestors are the foods to which we've become genetically adapted during the past $2^1/_2$ million years. And these same foods, or their modern-day equivalents, are the ones that should serve as a starting point for our optimal nutrition.

Although we live in a world of vast cities and complex technologies, each of us has a Stone Age genetic makeup. DNA studies from diverse ethnic groups around the world confirm that the present-day human genome is virtually identical to that of humans living forty thousand years ago.

Beginning some ten thousand years ago, people left behind the hunting and gathering way of life and began to sow and harvest the genetic forerunners of today's wheat and barley. Shortly thereafter, these early farmers domesticated farm animals (goats and sheep first, cows and pigs later). It took about five thousand years for the so-called Agricultural Revolution to spread from its origins in the Middle East to the farthest reaches of northern Europe and beyond.

But there has been very little time, evolutionarily speaking, for our bodies to adapt to this new way of eating. Although ten thousand years sounds historically remote, it is evolutionarily quite recent—only five hundred human generations have come and gone since agriculture began.

CHEESEBURGERS VERSUS BARBECUED BUFFALO

Cereal grains currently provide 50 percent of the protein consumed on the planet. Yet wild versions of this modern-day staple were rarely, if ever, consumed by hunter-gatherers and at best were considered foods to be consumed only to avoid starvation. Dairy products weren't part of humankind's original fare, either. (It's pretty difficult to catch a wild mammal, let alone milk one.) And except for rare treats of honey, refined sugars were not on the Stone Age menu. (By contrast, the typical American now consumes 152 pounds [69kg] of refined sugar per year.) Other foods that were not regular components of the hunter-gatherer diet include fatty meats, salt, yeast-containing foods, and legumes.

Obviously, the highly processed foods that now dominate the American diet were not part of the Paleolithic (Old Stone Age) meal plan. In fact, it's doubtful that hunter-gatherers would have recognized pizza, chips, French fries, ice cream, soda, and the like as food at all.

Lean game and fish were the staple foods in hunter-gatherer diets; consequently, the Paleolithic diet was much higher in protein than the typical U.S. diet. Because game is so lean on a calorie-by-calorie basis, it contains about two and a half times as much protein per serving as domestic meats. For instance, a 100-calorie serving of America's favorite meat—hamburger—contains a paltry 7.8 grams of protein. Compare that with 19.9 grams in an identical 100-calorie serving of roasted buffalo. Game is also healthier. It contains two to three times more cholesterol-lowering polyunsaturated fats and almost five times more omega-3 fatty acids than meat from grain-fed domestic livestock.

The carbohydrate content in the average hunter-gatherer diet was considerably lower than in the typical American diet of today as well. More importantly, it was made up almost entirely of wild fruits and vegetables. The total fat content was similar to or slightly higher than current U.S. figures; however, the types of fats were vastly different. The dominant fats in hunter-gatherer diets were healthful, cholesterol-lowering monounsaturated fats, which comprised about 50 percent of total fats consumed. By contrast, the typical U.S. diet has far fewer cholesterol-lowering mono- and polyunsaturated fats, more artery-clogging saturated fats and trans fats, and seven to ten times fewer heart-healthy omega-3 fatty acids than diets consumed by our hunter-gatherer forebears.

The key to the optimal human diet lies in the evolutionary wisdom of our hunter-gatherer past. The best high-protein options are fish (particularly fatty northern fish, such as salmon, halibut, mackerel, and herring), shellfish, grass-fed beef and pork, free-range chicken and turkey, rabbit, and any kind of game, either bought or hunted. The gastronomically adventurous can find buffalo, ostrich, emu, kangaroo, and venison at many upscale supermarkets and health food stores.

THE MISSING LINK BETWEEN DIET AND DISEASE

Contemporary hunter-gatherer tribes are almost completely free of the chronic diseases that plague Western civilization. Wild lean meats, organs, and fish are the mainstays of hunter-gatherer diets. How could these hunters and foragers be free of heart disease, high blood pressure and the sorts of cancers associated time and again with meat eating in the United States?

In the 1950s, when scientists were first unraveling the link between heart disease and diet, they found that saturated fat raised blood cholesterol levels and increased the risk for coronary heart disease. Dietary sources of saturated fat, such as fatty domestic meat, were deemed unhealthful, and rightly so. Unfortunately, the message the public and many nutrition professionals got was that meat was unhealthful and promoted heart disease and cancer. This notion was further ingrained by popular books written in the 1960s and '70s promoting vegetarian and vegan diets.

But it turns out that high amounts of animal protein, as predicted by the evolutionary template, are quite healthful for the human species. It's the saturated fat that can accompany that protein that causes the problems. The grains fed to most livestock turn healthful lean protein with a proper balance of good fats into a nutritional nightmare that promotes coronary heart disease and various types of cancer.

Consumption of lean meat actually lowers blood cholesterol levels and thereby reduces the risk of coronary heart disease. Consumption of lean animal protein elevates HDL cholesterol (the so-called "good" cholesterol) while reducing triglycerides, LDL cholesterol (the "bad" cholesterol), and total cholesterol. By contrast, low-fat, high-carbohydrate diets tend to elevate triglycerides and lower HDL cholesterol, thereby increasing the risk of coronary heart disease. High-carbohydrate diets also raise small, dense, LDL cholesterol—one of the most potent predictors for atherosclerosis and heart disease.

Other studies indicate that elevated dietary protein reduces the risk of stroke and hypertension and helps boost survival time for women with breast cancer. A high-protein diet also improves or normalizes insulin metabolism in type 2 diabetics. In other words, lean animal protein is good for us and saturated fat is not—exactly as predicted by our evolutionary template.

PUTTING IT ALL TOGETHER

The Paleo diet is the specific diet to which our species is genetically adapted. This program of eating was not designed by diet doctors, faddists, or nutritionists, but rather by Mother Nature's wisdom, acting through evolution and natural selection. The Paleo diet is based on extensive scientific research, examining the types and quantities of foods our hunter-gatherer ancestors ate. This nutritional plan is totally unlike those irresponsible, low-carbohydrate, high-fat, and fad diets that allow unlimited consumption of artery-clogging cheeses, bacon, butter, and fatty meats. Rather, the foundation of the Paleo diet is lean meat, seafood, and unlimited consumption of fresh fruits and veggies.

With readily available modern foods, the Paleo diet mimics the types of foods every single person on the planet ate prior to the Agricultural Revolution (a mere five hundred generations ago). These foods (fresh fruits, vegetables, lean meats, and seafood) are high in beneficial nutrients (soluble fiber, antioxidant vitamins, phytochemicals, omega-3s and monounsaturated fats, and low-glycemic carbohydrates) that promote good health, while they are low in the foods and nutrients (refined sugars and grains, saturated and trans fats, salt, high-glycemic carbohydrates, and processed foods) that frequently cause weight gain, cardiovascular disease, diabetes, and numerous other health problems. The Paleo diet encourages dieters to replace processed foods, dairy, and grain products with fresh fruits and vegetables—foods that are more nutritious than whole grains or dairy products.

You might consider the idea heretical that lean meat is healthful while whole grains and dairy products are not necessarily so. But the basis for this conclusion comes from overwhelming evolutionary evidence that is increasingly being substantiated by human, animal, and tissue studies. We all remain hunter-gatherers, displaced in time, yet still genetically adapted to a diet dominated by lean meats and fresh fruits and veggies.

6

Natural Gene Therapy

Vincent C. Giampapa, MD, FACS

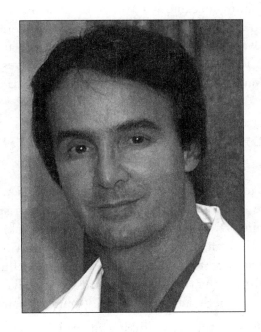

Vincent C. Giampapa is a founding member of the American Academy of Anti-Aging Medicine (A4M), past president of the American Board of Anti-Aging Medicine, a clinical assistant professor at the University of Medicine and Dentistry of New Jersey Medical Center in Newark, New Jersey, and director of the Giampapa Institute. Address: Skin & Body Clinic, 89 Valley Road, Montclair, NJ 07042. Tel: 973-746-3535. E-mail: giampapamd@aol.com. Website: www.skinbodyclinic.com

Over the past twenty years, the field of anti-aging medicine has evolved from simply incorporating lifestyle changes—such as diet, exercise, and vitamin administration as an anti-aging regimen—to sampling your individualized DNA and utilizing this information to create a personalized anti-aging program. This quantum leap of information has allowed the first generation of human beings to directly take charge of how they age and to be personally responsible for their ongoing health and longevity. I have witnessed these changes over the past two decades, and have been excited about helping people to significantly increase and improve the odds of their longevity.

Over the coming decade, a number of amazing new anti-aging therapies, based on personalized genetics, stem cell therapy, nanotechnology, and advances in drug-delivery systems, will allow us to add another dimension of health and longevity to our lives, provided we have taken advantage of the techniques and information now at our fingertips.

DNA: THE SOURCE OF HEALTH
AND OPTIMAL AGING

The blueprint for aging is contained within our DNA. With today's technology, we are able to sample our DNA with a small test that involves swabbing DNA from our buccal (inner cheek) cells. Within two weeks, this information can point to the key nutrients each of us needs, as individuals, to optimize five essential cellular processes directly related to aging. These five processes are glycation, inflammation, oxidation, methylation, and DNA (gene) repair.

1. *Glycation* refers to the cross-linking of proteins with sugar molecules at the cellular and genetic levels.

2. *Inflammation* refers to molecules released as a result of free radical damage; these molecules trigger inflammation in the tissues, causing pain, swelling, and dysfunction.

3. *Methylation* describes the activity at the genetic level that helps turn on or turn off our genes in the correct order.

4. *Oxidation* refers to the amount of free radical damage produced outside and inside the cell.

5. *DNA repair* reflects the efficiency of repairing damage to DNA from free radical attacks and environmental assaults; this is the most important gene function when it comes to keeping all cells functioning properly and staying healthy.

A brief look at the effects of calorie restriction (CR) over the last two or three years reveals that CR is the only scientifically documented way of slowing the aging process, as well as inhibiting the age-related diseases that occur with normal aging. For the first time, scientists have actually proven that we can affect the aging process in a positive way, improving the quality of our health and increasing our longevity.

Because restricting our calories by 30–40 percent in a calorie restriction program is extremely difficult for virtually all humans, I hypothesized that if we could mimic calorie restriction at the cellular level while reasonably altering our diet with fewer calories and fewer high-glycemic-index foods, we could perhaps create similar effects without the Spartan effort.

Calorie restriction offers a number of amazing effects, all documented in the scientific literature. These effects include:

- a reduction in free radical production
- a decrease in DNA damage and a concomitant increase in DNA repair
- a decrease in the loss of our stem cells, which are essential for cell regeneration
- a decrease in insulin production
- improvement of body composition
- a marked decrease in DNA damage overall, which lies at the root of virtually all accelerated aging

The most effective program that I found is called Age Management with personalized genetic health testing.

PERSONALIZED GENETIC HEALTH

The personalized genetic health program, which I have been utilizing over the last seven years, involves taking a sample of a person's genetic material with an eye toward assessing the five essential cellular processes listed above. The goal is to mimic calorie restriction at the cellular level, so we can alter our gene expression patterns in ways that help us live longer and stay stronger.

THE IDEAL CALORIE RESTRICTION PRESCRIPTION MEDICATION: METFORMIN

A large amount of research over the past decade has documented that the diabetic medication Metformin not only lowers blood sugar by improving insulin receptor sensitivity, but also interacts with the same group of genes that are positively affected by calorie restriction. As it turns out, prescribing Metformin in microdoses for nondiabetic people boosts insulin sensitivity in these nondiabetics, and actually alters the five groups of gene categories mentioned above in much the same way that calorie restriction operates.

Other prescription medications can further enhance this effect. For instance, COX-2 inhibitors—in a natural form from hops extract and/or in prescription medications—can improve inflammatory gene function. Drugs that are involved in antioxidation, like Deprenyl, can promote the antioxidant action of intrinsic antioxidants like superoxide dismutase, catalase, and glutathione peroxidase. Other prescription medications that figure in methylation, as well as DNA repair, also fast-track the program.

ADULT STEM CELL THERAPY

Also available today are stem cell therapies that allow us to both harvest and store our adult stem cells. One of the key factors in aging is now recognized as a decrease in the number of stem cells, as well as a change in gene expression patterns within the stem cells. The number of stem cells is directly related to our ability to restore our somatic, or body, cells as they wear out or are injured by infection and/or disease. Our newfound ability to extract and store adult stem cells will revolutionize the anti-aging industry in the future. Why? Because we can then utilize these stem cells in large numbers as we grow older, and we will be able to alter those genes—and insert new ones—to mimic the effects of calorie restriction and address issues of aging at the cellular level.

Certain compounds and supplements have already been formulated to help release stem cells when they are needed to help enhance surgical recovery and regeneration. These compounds are available through injection at anti-aging centers.

Another strategy I use with my patients revolves around gene expression modification.

GEMs

GEMs, or gene expression modifiers, are compounds that have the unique ability to demethylate promoter regions—the start segments—of our genes and remethylate other areas of our genome, actually altering or turning on and off specific genes and groups of genes. These gene expression modifiers are naturally occurring compounds produced in the liver and other tissues. Recently discovered and synthesized, they can be utilized as part of an ongoing anti-aging program.

GEMs turn off oncogenes and turn back on tumor suppressor genes. They also improve skin texture and quality, plus cholesterol levels, as well as bolstering other key functions that become less efficient as aging progresses.

I have combined all the above information and biotechnology into the new anti-aging program that I myself follow, as do many of my patients at the Giampapa Institute.

My program includes the following:

1. Personalized genetic health gene testing to document genetic deficiencies.

2. The use of a core nutrition supplement and gene-directed nutraceuticals.

3. The use of category-specific prescription compounds to further boost the supplement program.

4. A program of approximately four months of gene expression modifiers to repair DNA damage and reprogram genes prior to harvest.

5. The harvesting and storage of reprogrammed adult stem cells for future use for both regenerative and cosmetic applications.

6. An environmental lifestyle modification program, which focuses on diet, exercise, and mind state.

IT'S NOT JUST YOUR GENES . . .

We have finally realized that it is not just our genes that dictate our future health and longevity, but it is the environment in which they are placed. In my personal anti-aging program, I include all the above approaches in a comprehensive personalized program, not only for myself but for prospective patients and people who are intimately concerned with taking charge of their own future health and longevity.

Simple at-home urine tests can help monitor DNA damage and free radical levels, the two key biomarkers or actual lab tests that indicate the level of the cellular aging process.

IN SUMMARY

At present, we have the science, technology, and laboratory diagnostic testing to markedly improve the quality of our health, the quality of our time, and our longevity. This approach will give us the ability to maintain our health at the level of our DNA, and to maintain DNA function and integrity long enough to benefit from the future technologies that will arrive within the next seven to ten years.

For the first time in history, we have this information and power at our fingertips. It will allow us to take control of our own health and to perhaps markedly extend what were once thought to be the limits of human health and longevity.

7

A Natural Anti-Aging Compound

Ann Louise Gittleman, PhD, CNS, ND, MS

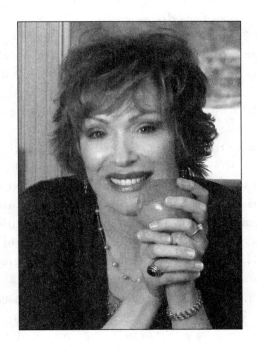

Ann Louise Gittleman is one of the foremost experts on nutrition and healthy eating. Her books include the best-selling *Fat Flush Plan,* as well as *Before the Change, Beyond Pritikin,* and *Eat Fat, Lose Weight.* E-mail: sgittleman@annlouise.com. Website: www.annlouise.com

My roots have always been very holistic. Ever since I heard the name *Adele Davis* way back as a sophomore at Connecticut College in New London, Connecticut, I have been bitten by the nutrition bug. I believed then, as I do now, that health and longevity are within our grasp as long as we are looking in the right places. I experimented a lot in those early days. When many of my contemporaries were dabbling with mind-altering substances, I began searching for the fountain of youth—a one-stop-shop natural health solution to deal with the most urgent concerns of aging that my contemporaries and I seemed destined to face—arthritis, loss of memory, chronic pain, depression, and loss of sex drive.

Diet by diet, my personal health odyssey and longevity journey transformed me into a vegetarian, vegan, raw-foods aficionado, and macrobiotic devotee—only to learn the hard way that what seemed like the "right" and "responsible" way to eat for vitality and longevity never seemed to work for my type-A, sympathetic-dominant personality.

When I became the director of nutrition at the Pritikin Longevity Center in Santa Monica, California in the early '80s, I came to the realization that while diet was an important element in achieving total health, there had to be something more. In my position at Pritikin, I had the opportunity to speak with a number of celebrities, CEOs, and artists—all of whom had traveled throughout the world. In the course of taking their health and diet histories, many of these distinguished individuals casually mentioned that they had routinely traveled to Romania for Dr. Ana Aslan's procaine therapy, known as Gerovital H-3 (or GH-3).

I became intrigued by the glowing reports of the extraordinary results obtained from this therapy and soon began my own research into this most amazing anti-aging remedy. From my studies and review of medical articles, books, and consultations with my Pritikin clients, I learned that patients receiving procaine therapy showed a much deeper capacity for joy in everyday life, experienced relief from anxiety and depression; had increased intellectual and physical vigor; and experienced less stiffness, better skin, enhanced hair and nail growth, fewer brown spots and skin abnormalities, and faster healing of accidental fractures. Consistently, people spoke about being able to sleep through the night (finally) and waking up feeling alert, as well as having a better memory. They all raved about their ability to cope with stress better in as short a period as two weeks, mind you. Many individuals even weaned themselves off prescription drugs with their doctor's blessing.

TURN BACK THE CLOCK
WITH THE ROMANIAN ANTI-AGING MIRACLE

As is true with most great discoveries, procaine, the primary active ingredient in GH-3, was discovered by accident. In 1949, Dr. Ana Aslan of the National Geriatric Institute in Bucharest, Romania began to use procaine for its anesthetic properties with her elderly arthritis patients. To her amazement, Aslan's patients not only became pain-free but they also demonstrated dramatic mental and physical improvements. Many reported an enhanced sex drive, too!

Aslan basically believed that procaine worked its "magic" by repairing old and damaged cell membranes so they could absorb nutrients more efficiently. Her observations prompted her to organize clinical trials that studied the impact of procaine on individuals between thirty-eight and sixty-two. There were 15,000 patients included in these preliminary trials, with more than 400 doctors and over 150 clinics participating—a very impressive double-blind trial if ever there was one.

The research team discovered that about 70 percent of Aslan's patients never got sick, the death rate from the Aslan group was five times lower than the placebo group, patients were less prone to infections, and joint mobility was enhanced in over 50 percent of the cases. Diseases like depression, chronic fatigue, Parkinson's, heart disease, migraine headaches, arthritis, hypertension, poor circulation, and osteoporosis were improved with GH-3. Even liver spots were said to disappear and patients' original hair color returned.

As time went on, there were over five hundred laboratory studies conducted by gerontologists and leading physicians from all over the world. One finding, in particular, began to emerge that explained the extraordinary rejuvenating powers of GH-3. It was discovered that GH-3 had the ability to inhibit and balance the buildup in the brain of a particular enzyme, known as monoamine oxidase (MAO). Researchers believe that after the age of forty-five, the body starts to make higher and higher levels of this enzyme, which replaces other hormones, producing depression and premature aging. As a natural tranquilizer without side effects, Gerovital H-3 was on its way into the U.S. market, or so it should have been.

THE POLITICS OF HEALTH

Sadly, throughout the 1960s, Gerovital was kept off the U.S. market by obstacles placed in its way by federal regulations. When Mike Wallace of *60 Minutes* did a piece on the product in 1972, the secret was out. Thousands of people began treatment in Romania for the so-called Fountain of Youth.

World leaders, like Charles de Gaulle, Ho Chi Minh, Mao Tse-Tung, and John F. Kennedy, were purported users. Hollywood stars, including Lena Horne, Charles Bronson, Greta Garbo, and Marlene Dietrich, also flocked to Dr. Aslan's treatments.

Right around the time when I began to hear about GH-3, in the early 1980s, the Romanian sources were beginning to dry up. There were also concerns that the market was being inundated with ineffective and cheap imitations.

THE NEXT GENERATION GH-3: ULTRA H-3™

Inspired by the research, I was offered the opportunity to research and design the next generation GH-3, which was named Ultra H-3™. As I will soon enter a brand-new decade of life, my overriding concern for this product is to ensure the most efficient way in which it can target brain health (now that I am older, my priorities have changed, too).

As we now know, as people grow older the brain undergoes macroscopic, microscopic, biochemical, and electrophysiological changes. Cognitive function begins its decline and age-related senility and depression begin their rise. Since I was aware of the MAO connection in all of this, I knew that it was important not only to balance the MAOs for improved mental clarity (which Ultra H-3™ does accomplish) but also to make sure that circulation to the brain is enhanced. The addition of gingko biloba and bilberry extracts to the Ultra H-3™ formula ensures the targeted delivery of nutrients through the blood/brain barrier.

The new Ultra H-3™ is also a patent-protected procaine product, which is considered 100 percent bioavailable. It lasts about fifteen times longer than the original injectable product and is also about six times stronger. It's almost like a powerful yet gentle adaptogenic herb—the product seems to provide whatever your body requires or is lacking.

Most individuals start with one or two tablets in the morning and follow up with another one or two in the afternoon about six to eight hours apart to ensure adequate blood levels.

Each tablet of Ultra H-3™ contains 100 mg of procaine hydrochloride. As it breaks down, it releases its natural constituents of para-aminobenzoic acid (PABA) and diethylaminoethanol (DEAE). PABA is a stimulant to the beneficial intestinal bacteria that aid in the production of vitamins K and B_1, and folic acid. DEAE is involved in the production of acetylcholine, so vital to the nerve and brain synapses. I find that both these ingredients act like natural muscle relaxants and have antihistamine properties as well. In addition to the procaine itself, Ultra H-3™ contains a matrix of ascorbic acid, citric acid, niacin, folic acid, biotin, and magnesium, which helps to protect the procaine from breaking down too quickly in the system—all in a base of gingko biloba and bilberry extracts to optimize circulation throughout the body.

Available through UNI KEY, at 1-800-888-4353, this product can be taken with your other dietary supplements. As a matter of fact, I believe that all your other vitamins, minerals, enzymes, and digestive aids will be assimilated and absorbed more effectively and efficiently while taking Ultra H-3™.

LOOKING TOWARD THE FUTURE

I am sure there are many additional all-natural ways to reverse the aging process that you will have the pleasure of discovering by reading this wonderful book. The best news of all is that the "fountain of youth" really does exist, although it may be different for each one of us. For me, finding GH-3, and later helping to develop its successor, Ultra H-3™, was a blessing. It is my fervent hope that you will be blessed, too, whatever your path may be to the Fountain.

8

Physical Fitness as Part of Longevity

Robert Goldman, MD, PhD, DO, FAASP

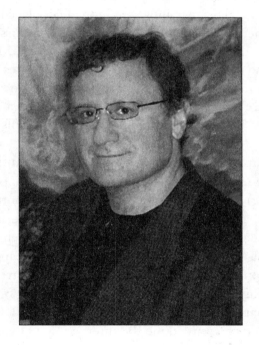

Robert Goldman is chairman of the American Academy of Anti-Aging Medicine (A4M). Address: 1510 West Montana Street, Chicago, IL 60614. Tel: 773-528-4333. Website: www.worldhealth.net

As a physician cofounder of the American Academy of Anti-Aging Medicine (A4M) with Dr. Ronald Klatz (see his chapter, starting on p. 00) and as A4M chairman, I have the privilege of traveling to more than twenty nations a year with the specific objective of raising awareness about, and increasing the adoption of, anti-aging and regenerative medicine. My frequent trips overseas have launched a number of initiatives that promote innovative approaches to address the swelling aging population in nations around the world. In expanding the reach of anti-aging and regenerative medicine, A4M adopts the Olympic model for global expansion. We aim to develop strong international partnerships with individuals placed in prominent positions in their respective nations' medical commissions; governmental bodies, including the Medical Commission of the European Parliament; and academic and research-based affiliates and universities. In doing so, we have garnered strong participation among nations in Europe and Asia, as well as in South and Central America, and Canada. Today, 15 percent of A4M's membership hails from outside U.S. borders.

I consider fitness to be a universal and leading anti-aging intervention. I cofounded the National Academy of Sports Medicine (www.nasm.org), the global leader in certification, continuing education, solutions, and tools for health, fitness, sports performance, and sports medicine professionals, serving over 100,000 members in eighty countries. As a black belt in karate, a Chinese weapons expert, a world-champion athlete with over twenty world strength records (including listings in the *Guinness Book of World Records*), I was inducted into the National Fitness Hall of Fame in 2007. In 2001, Juan Antonio Samaranch awarded me the International Olympic Committee tribute diploma for contributions to the development of sport and Olympism.

My concept of anti-aging medicine considers the specialty to be the next generation of sports medicine. In sports medicine, physicians aim to keep athletes in peak physical and mental condition, to maximize their performance in competition. Anti-aging medicine seeks to keep people in top physical and mental shape as they age.

MAKE HEALTHY CHOICES

Adopt the Anti-Aging Lifestyle

Kay-Tee Khaw from Cambridge University (United Kingdom), and colleagues, followed twenty thousand men and women, ages forty-five to seventy-nine, for thirteen years. They questioned the study subjects about their lifestyles and conducted blood tests to measure vitamin C levels (an indicator of daily fruit and vegetable intake). Those study subjects with the lowest number of healthy behaviors were four times more likely to die, usually from cardiovascular disease. The team found that study participants with the lowest healthy lifestyle scores had the same risk of dying as a person with the highest healthy lifestyle scores who was fourteen years older. The lifestyle change with the biggest benefit was smoking cessation, associated with an 80 percent improvement in life span. The second most significant change was associated with increased consumption of fresh fruits and vegetables. Ranked third was moderate drinking; fourth, staying physically active, rounded out the four most beneficial lifestyle choices to extend one's life span.

This study validates the anti-aging lifestyle, hallmarks of which include the following:

- not smoking

- eating five or more servings of fresh fruits and vegetables a day

- moderate alcohol consumption

- regular aerobic exercise.

Not only does the anti-aging lifestyle extend life span, it prolongs *health span*, the length of time that we are able to live productively and independently. Because this study found that life span extension via these four lifestyle choices held true regardless of age, sex, and socio-economic status, it clearly demonstrates the applicability of the anti-aging lifestyle across a broad base of the population.

GET QUALITY SLEEP

As a frequent overseas traveler, I have devised a practical, tried-and-true program that often helps me boost the quality of my sleep. Highlights include:

1. Practice good sleep hygiene:

   • Where you sleep directly impacts how well you sleep: Create a sleeping environment that is comfortable in temperature, sans distracting lighting and sounds, and serene.

   • Don't become overstimulated: Keep appliances that emit electromagnetic fields (televisions, cell phones, etc.) at least ten feet (3m) away from the bed.

   • If you are allergic to airborne agents, remove plants and humidifiers (both can be sources of mold), don't let pets into your bedroom (sources of dander), and encase your mattress, box spring, blankets, and pillows (havens for dust mites) in allergy-barrier covers.

2. Eat for sleep: Starchy foods like breads, pastas, potatoes, and milk products help promote sleep. They prompt your brain to generate the sleep-inducing neurochemical serotonin.

3. Herbs help: For some people, a modest dose of valerian root, kava, chamomile, or lavender oil speed up the trip to dreamland.

4. Avoid certain medications: Check with your physician to verify whether any prescription and/or over-the-counter products you take may be interfering with your ability to fall asleep. Blood pressure medicines, decongestants, nicotine, caffeine, diet pills, and some cold/cough remedies are frequent culprits.

5. Lower your body temperature: You reach sleep once your body temperature dips. A warm bath or shower before bedtime makes it easier for your body to cool down and the time to reach dreamland shorter.

6. Take a power nap: Just twenty minutes of restful slumber during a hectic day not only rejuvenates your thinking, but can make it easier for you to sleep at night.

FITNESS AS A UNIVERSAL AND LEADING ANTI-AGING INTERVENTION

Obesity is the second-leading cause of preventable deaths the world over. According to the American Obesity Association, about 69 million Americans are overweight and 51 million are obese. These numbers have been rising steadily, meaning that 61 percent of U.S. adults twenty years of age and over are overweight, and 26 percent are obese. Annually, overweight/obesity causes at least 300,000 excess deaths in the United States, burdening the nation with a health care tab of more than $100 billion each year. Medical risks associated with obesity include type 2 diabetes, gout, hypertension, osteoarthritis, cardiovascular disease, sleep apnea, high cholesterol, cancers, gallbladder disease, impaired respiratory function, and—in women—an increased incidence of varicose veins, asthma, and hemorrhoids.

One of the most potent forms of anti-aging medicine is exercise. Substantial health benefits occur with regular physical activity that is aerobic in nature (such as thrity to sixty minutes of brisk walking five or more days of the week). Additional health benefits can be gained through greater amounts of physical activity, but even small amounts of activity are healthier than a sedentary lifestyle. Regular exercise in middle age can help men and women prolong their physical prowess as they grow older.

While aerobic exercise is important to keep weight within a healthy range and bolster the cardiovascular system, strength training is just as important. Strength training, also referred to as resistance training, enables men and women at any age to improve their overall health and fitness by increasing muscular strength, endurance, and bone density. This particular type of physical activity also enhances insulin sensitivity and glucose metabolism. Strength training recommendations include:

- Perform exercises two or more days a week.

- Use handheld light dumbbells, free weights, machines, or resistance bands, or no weights at all.

- If weights are used, start with one to two pounds (.5–1kg) and gradually increase the weight over time.

- Perform exercises that involve the major muscle groups (arms, shoulders, chest, abdomen, back, hips, and legs) and exercises that enhance grip strength.

- Perform eight to fifteen repetitions of each exercise, then perform a second set.

- Do not hold your breath during strength exercises.

- Rest between sets.

- Avoid locking the joints in your arms and legs.

- Stretch after completing all exercises.

- Stop if you feel pain at any time.

- Conduct strength training only after consulting with a qualified medical professional.

Studies show that even men and women in their nineties who took up weight training increased muscle mass and strengthened bones, key improvements in preventing falls and injuries and encouraging continued independent living. Yet, only 11 percent of older adults follow strength training recommendations. The vast majority of older adults are missing opportunities to improve their health through strength training. Fortunately, the fix is simple to make.

A study conducted by researchers at the University of Michigan should inspire readers in their fifties and sixties to become physically active—especially if you have conditions or habits that endanger your heart, like diabetes, high blood pressure, or smoking. In this study, which involved 9,611 older adults, those who were regularly active in their fifties and sixties were 35 percent less likely to die in the next eight years than those who were sedentary. The reduction in the risk of early death was achieved in study participants who engaged in very moderate physical activity: the reduction was seen among those who took leisurely walks, gardened, or went dancing a few times a week. Even those who were obese had a lower risk of dying if they were regularly active. The researchers observed that "We found across all ranges of cardiovascular risk, everybody got a benefit from regular activity, but the biggest absolute benefit, the biggest reduction in deaths, was among high risk people." Continuing, the researchers remarked that, in people who have cardiovascular issues, "the risk of remaining sedentary" is far greater than "the risk of having an acute problem brought on by exercise."

Physical exercise has also now been shown to help maintain our mental health. Physically active adults have sharper concentration skills, which may help maintain memory and combat dementia. In a study by researchers at Northwestern University's Feinberg School of Medicine in Chicago, Dr. Susan Benloucif and colleagues found that sedentary lifestyles directly contribute to the decline in cognitive abilities and quality of sleep as we age. Twelve men and women, ages sixty-seven to eighty-six, who were functionally independent, participated in a two-week study involving a regimen of thirty minutes of mild physical activity, thirty minutes of social interaction, and a final thirty minutes of mild to moderate physical activity. Sessions began with warm-up stretching and mild to moderate physical activity (walking, stationary upper- and lower-body exercises). The final period of mild to moderate physical activity included rapid walking, calisthenics, or dancing. A ten-minute cooldown concluded the ninety-minute regimen. At the end of the two-week period, all participants demonstrated a 4–6 percent improvement in cognitive performance, and improved sleep quality (including deeper sleep and fewer awakenings).

Exercise is a universally accessible anti-aging modality. It's never too early—or too late—to start a regimen of physical activity, and the benefits of doing so are wide ranging for you and your loved ones.

CONCLUSION

Thanks to current and future advancements in anti-aging and regenerative medicine, the American Academy of Anti-Aging Medicine projects that the human life span will reach upwards of 125 years and beyond by the year 2049. I expect to live at least 125 productive, healthy, and vital years. Adopt the anti-aging lifestyle, get quality sleep, and engage in regular physical activity, and you just might accomplish the same.

9

Prolonging Healthy and Productive Life

Abram Hoffer, PhD, MD, FRCP(C)

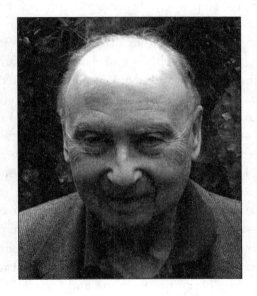

Abram Hoffer is one of the pioneers of orthomolecular, or nutritional, medicine, and the author of many scientific papers and books, including *Adventures in Psychiatry, Hoffer's Laws of Natural Nutrition,* and *Vitamin B3 and Schizophrenia.* He and his colleagues developed the first nutritional treatment of schizophrenia (vitamins B_3 and C) and discovered the cholesterol-lowering benefits of niacin (one of the forms of vitamin B_3). He is president of the Orthomolecular Vitamin Information Centre, Inc. Website: www.orthomolecularvitamincentre.com

never thought I would search for the Holy Grail—eternal youth—nor do I think it will ever be found. But looking back at my career over the past fifty years, it's odd how the research I did gradually involved me more and more in the search for better health and longevity.

I had gotten my PhD in agricultural biochemistry and later my MD. During my early career as a vitamin control analyst in cereal grains, I became aware of the importance of the newly discovered and synthesized vitamins. The United States had just mandated the fortification of flour with a few B vitamins, and within about two years a major pandemic called pellagra was brought under control. This probably did more to enrich and extend life and to prevent mental illness than any other previous public health measure. The two main outcomes of pellagra were psychosis and death. Small amounts of vitamin B_3 cured the psychosis and people no longer were dying from this deficiency disease. No action by psychiatric theory and practice has ever equaled this amazing public health measure. During the great pellagra pandemics, up to one-third of mental hospital admissions in the southeastern United States were psychotic pellagrins who could not be distinguished clinically from those with schizophrenia.

In 1950 I became director of psychiatric research in the Province of Saskatchewan and selected schizophrenia as our main target. Half of our six thousand patients in three institutions were psychotic, with no hope of ever getting well. The adrenochrome hypothesis of schizophrenia (based on the idea that oxidized adrenaline causes hallucinations), developed by Humphry Osmond and myself, led to our use of vitamin B_3 as a treatment. There are two forms of this vitamin: niacin and niacinamide. We had to be certain that long-term use of these vitamins would be safe. They are safe. I have been taking niacin for the past fifty-two years—I should be in the *Guinness Book of World Records*. In searching for toxic side effects, we ran across none, and instead discovered many beneficial side effects, such as the normalizing effect of niacin (but not of niacinamide) on blood lipid levels. It is the world's gold standard for lowering total cholesterol, for elevating HDL, for decreasing triglycerides, for decreasing Lipo A, as a major anti-inflammatory substance and, not surprisingly, in decreasing mortality and extending life.

In 1954, my mother complained to me that she was losing her memory, could not see well from her left eye, and had arthritis in her fingers; I saw the Heberden's nodes (bony growths). Knowing I could not help her, I gave her niacin, which was safe, as I thought it would have a positive placebo effect. To my amazement, three months later she was normal, her nodes were flattening, and her vision had returned, as had her memory. She lived many more years and wrote two books before she died at age eighty-seven. I became convinced that pathological aging was not inevitable.

I began to take niacin myself, 1 gram after each of three meals. I wanted to experience the niacin flush so I could better explain this to my patients. Two weeks later, my bleeding, swollen, and boggy gums, which had troubled me for a long time, were clear and my gums were firm. I began to wonder whether this was due to accelerated healing from the niacin. This led to my suggestion to Professor Rudl Altschul, chair, Department of Anatomy, who was studying arteriosclerosis in rabbits, to see if niacin would help heal the intima of the arteries, which he suggested was a major factor. I gave him 1 pound (.5kg) of pure niacin. He did not study its effect on the intima but instead found that it lowered cholesterol in his rabbits; later we found the same result in humans. I decided to see what long-term niacin use would do for me.

Today, nearly fifty years later, I still wonder but I will not stop it. My journey began from niacin and vitamin C, and led to the influence of hypoglycemia, to other vitamins and minerals, essential fatty acids, and eventually to orthomolecular medicine. My present personal program for improving one's chances for healthy aging is based on this experience and on the over ten thousand patients I have seen during my career as a physician. One of my patients died at age 112, the oldest person in Saskatchewan at that time, and perhaps in Canada. She had been cross-country skiing until age 110 and was photographed playing a piano duet with her great-grandson before she died. She took niacin for forty-two years.

FOOD AND THE WAYS TO EAT

I advised my patients to follow a few simple food rules: (1) Avoid foods that you know make you sick; these are foods to which they are allergic. Also avoid foods that are going to make you sick; these include all the pure sugars, processed carbohydrates to excess, and processed foods that have lost too much of their nutrient quality due to the processing. A good rule is to avoid any food preparation that contains added sugar. Usually these foods also contain most of the other additives that are allowed in our foods. (2) If possible, eat three meals each day, starting with a healthy, protein-rich breakfast; I do not consider a doughnut and coffee a healthy breakfast. I also listen to my daughter Miriam, a retired dietitian from Women's College Hospital in Toronto. I avoid all dairy products, eggs, wheat, oats, peanuts, coconut, pecans, and sugar because they make *me* sick.

VITAMINS

I do not consider any one vitamin superior to any other. They are all essential. Any deficiency of a particular nutrient will increase ill health and decrease life span. For any person, the most important nutrient is the one that is missing. Since it can be very difficult to determine which of the B vitamins may be lacking, it's a wise policy to take them all in the form of one of the many B-complex preparations that are available. I prefer the B-complex 50s or B-complex 100s, one daily.

However, many people have developed a need for greater amounts of the vitamins than can be provided even with these B-complex preparations. They have a vitamin dependency. They should take increased doses of the B vitamins, as they are dependent on some of them. I suspect that when proper searches are made, patients will be found who are dependent on every known vitamin. Fewer patients will have double dependencies. I have suggested that Huntington's disease is caused by a double deficiency of niacin and vitamin E. Several of my patients with HD recovered on large doses of these two nutrients. I doubt that triple-dependency babies will ever be born alive.

MY PERSONAL PROGRAM

This is the program I have been following, but I do not recommend this for everyone. We are much too individualistic for one program to fit all; each of us must determine for ourselves what works best for us.

This can be used as a model, but it should not to be followed slavishly. It is based on the principles of orthomolecular medicine, a wonderful and accurate term presented to us all as a gift by Linus Pauling, two-time Nobel Prize winner. It is best to start as early as possible, but it never too late to start.

- Vitamin A: 30,000 IU daily
- Niacin: 1 gram three times daily
- Vitamin C: 1 gram twice daily
- B-complex 100: one daily
- Folic acid: 5 mg daily
- Vitamin D: 6,000 IU daily
- Vitamin E: 400 IU twice daily
- Selenium: 200 mcg daily
- Calcium citrate: 660 mg daily
- Magnesium: 330 mg daily
- Zinc citrate: 50 mg daily
- Salmon oil: 1 gram three times daily
- Coenzyme Q_{10}: 100 mg three times daily
- N-acetyl cysteine: 1 gram three times daily
- Alpha-lipoic acid: 200 mg three times daily

Niacin

This is my favorite, but not the most important vitamin. The amount needed varies tremendously; most niacin-dependent people will need 500–3,000 mg three times daily, always to be taken after meals. No one should take niacin until they have read about it and the flush it causes when it is first started. There is no point in asking your doctors, since they probably know less about it than you do. In my book with Harold D. Foster, called *Feel Better, Live Longer with Vitamin B$_3$*, we provide a detailed description of the many valuable properties of this vitamin. The National Coronary Drug Study showed that men who had suffered one coronary and were given niacin lived two years longer than those on controls or other drugs.

Vitamin C

Very few people eat as many vegetables containing this vitamin as do our gorilla cousins in zoos, as well as in the wild. The optimum amount varies enormously. However, I find that unless there are special needs, such as for colds, infections, or cancer, 3–6 grams per day is adequate. The upper limit is determined by bowel tolerance.

Vitamin D

The only time I got a lot of vitamin D was when I was working on our farm during those hot, dry, Saskatchewan days, I didn't lather myself with sunscreen, and my shirt was off because of the heat. I did not develop any skin cancer, but I did get a great tan. Now I depend on the six little pills I take each day, but I get no tan.

Vitamin E

Antioxidants like this, which counter fat-soluble free radicals, are also useful.

Coenzyme Q$_{10}$

This essential compound should be included with the vitamins, as we cannot make enough when we are sick or get old. And drugs, particularly the statins, prevent the body from making it. It is an essential component of factor A in the respiratory chain, in combination with vitamin B$_3$.

N-Acetyl Cysteine and Alpha-lipoic Acid

These two sulfur-containing antioxidants increase the production of glutathione peroxidase. N-acetyl cysteine is a very powerful, safe antioxidant. Alpha-lipoic acid protects the liver against toxic substances. I take them both, following information from Jack Challem that they can be helpful in controlling glaucoma. I was placed on glaucoma watch, but after a few months on these two substances I was taken off glaucoma watch and my ocular pressure is normal.

Selenium

I am one of the few people who are not deficient in this very important trace element. I am sorry for the people infected with the HIV virus who have to take the toxic antiretroviral drugs when they do have a choice of taking selenium and three amino acids—glutamine, cysteine, and tryptophan—with much better recoveries and no side effects. Every additional vaccine trial, costing Bill Gates millions and affecting thousands of people, has been proven not to be effective. But the vaccine establishment remains optimistic and expects in ten years that one will be found. Money for the Holy Grail, the magic pill, the omnipotent vaccine rolls on and on. Selenium is way too cheap.

PHYSICAL ACTIVITY

I keep as active as I can at age ninety-one. Activity includes doing all the things one has to do to keep alive, like shopping, walking, going to the office, climbing stairs, going to the mailbox and exercise, which I do under the guidance of my personal, tough, friendly trainer. I do about forty-five minutes every morning and an additional hour with her twice each week. She is getting me ready for the centenarian Olympics. I walk between 1,500 and 2,500 steps daily. Anyone who expects me to do 10,000 steps a day is nuts.

AVOID DRUGS

Linus Pauling advised people *not* to consult their doctors. He meant one should work with orthomolecular doctors. I am very careful about whom I consult and seriously censor whatever they tell me. This is a luxury most people do not have. My doctors are good. My son is a professor of medicine at McGill University. That is great protection.

TAKE CHARGE

You and your medical and health advisors are real partners in the enterprise of keeping you well. Don't leave all the responsibility up to them. Unfortunately, you will have to read all about orthomolecular therapy on your own, or travel far to find an orthomolecular therapist. So far this very valuable treatment is available only to the rich, and to those dedicated to better health. Doctors have not heard of it, psychiatrists totally reject it, and medical insurance plans will not cover it.

10

Picking the Right Supplements

Ronald L. Hoffman, MD, CNS

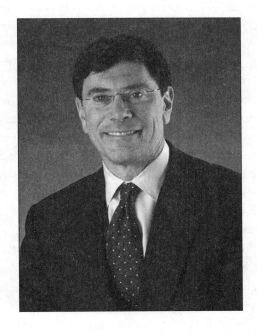

Ronald Hoffman is medical director of the Hoffman Center, a nutrition-ally oriented medical clinic in New York City. He is the author of *How to Talk with Your Doctor, Alternative Cures that Really Work,* and many other books. Address: The Hoffman Center, 776 Sixth Avenue, Suite 4B, New York, NY 10001. Tel: 212-779-1744. Website: www.drhoffman.com

Selecting supplements for your own personal program is lot like creating a properly diversified personal investment portfolio. The analogy is appropriate. Both investment and nutrition are evidence-based sciences, but they are forward-looking and hence inexact. Today's best bet is merely an extension of present knowledge.

Both investment and supplement portfolios can be conservative, or they can be highly speculative. The potential returns—and risks—rise accordingly. There are some whose sophistication and risk tolerance extend no further than Centrum and tax-free muni bonds. Others gravitate to exotic hedge funds and elaborate nutritional "cocktails."

Additionally, experience modifies our choices—we add or shed investments according to their performance or the latest data. Those who buck the wisdom of "The Street" or of conventional medicine do so at their own peril, but the rewards can be huge for great visionaries.

And finally, to complete the analogy, yes—there is fraud and no shortage of unscrupulous advisors in the realm of finance as well as in nutrition, and while professional accreditation is a partial safeguard, there is no substitute for an advisor with a great track record, who makes accurate predications and is untainted by a history of conspicuous failures.

Why take all these supplements? Recently, the press has been touting a spate of studies that purport to show that taking supplements is at best a waste of time, at worst dangerous. What are the facts?

A study published in the peer-reviewed *Nutrition Journal* (October 24, 2007) reveals that people who used multiple supplements—taking, on average, seventeen different supplements daily for at least twenty years—were in overall better health than both nonsupplement users and individuals who only consumed a single multivitamin/multimineral supplement. This first-ever study on long-term users of multiple dietary supplements found them comparatively to have markedly better health.

As a group, they were 73 percent less likely to have diabetes and 39 percent less likely to have elevated blood pressure than nonusers. Also, this group was less likely to have suboptimal blood nutrient concentrations, and more likely to have favorable levels of key biomarkers, including serum homocysteine, C-reactive protein, high-density-lipoprotein (HDL) cholesterol (the so-called "good" cholesterol), and triglycerides than either nonusers or multivitamin/multimineral users. Perhaps for the first time, this study underscored the importance of taking a full portfolio of nutritional supplements.

So here are some core recommendations for creating your own nutritional portfolio.

START WITH A GOOD MULTI

There are multis and there are multis. It is virtually impossible to incorporate a full spectrum of quality basic nutrients in a single "once-a-day," so forget those. The best multis require a daily dose of at least two, and sometimes up to six tablets or capsules a day, because minerals like calcium and magnesium are bulky.

Your multi should include all the major vitamins and minerals in amounts that *exceed* the government's recommended daily allowance (RDA). Beware of multis that contain token amounts of critical nutrients just to create the false impression that they are comprehensive.

When it comes to multis, beware of gimmicks. Some multis contain "herbal blends" or tiny amounts of special nutrients like coenzyme Q_{10} or alpha-lipoic acid. Such nutrients are valuable, but must be present in significant amounts and are best taken separately at effective therapeutic doses.

ADD ANTIOXIDANTS

A concerted campaign has been underway to debunk the importance of antioxidants. A few new meta-analyses have cherry-picked research to show that antioxidants are overrated or even harmful. But many of these studies were done in artificial settings, on sick or dying patients, for short durations, and with low-quality synthetic ingredients. Antioxidants do work, and thousands of scientific studies continue to support their efficacy for the prevention of a variety of degenerative diseases. Some recent studies have suggested that, far from being dangerous at high doses, certain antioxidants like vitamin E may have to be used at even higher doses.

Add mixed carotenoids (not just beta carotene): 10,000–15,000 IU;

vitamin E (mixed tocopherols, rich in gamma tocopherol): 400 IU; vitamin C: 500 mg at least three times daily; chelated zinc: 30 mg per day; and chelated selenium: 200 mcg per day.

And don't forget "special" antioxidants like alpha-lipoic acid and N-acetyl cysteine (NAC). These antioxidants have powerful systemic protective effects on the brain, the lungs, the heart, the liver, and the kidneys, and even have been proposed as key anti-aging nutrients. Take alpha-lipoic acid at 300 mg twice daily, and NAC at 500 mg twice daily.

GET AN OIL CHANGE

A basic nutrient that is an essential part of a core nutritional portfolio is omega-3. EPA and DHA from fish oil (but not present in vegetable omega-3s like flax oil) fight inflammation, heart disease, cancer, and literally help make you smarter and balance your mood. Look for pharmaceutical-grade fish oil in capsules or liquid, and consume 2–8 grams (2 teaspoonsful) per day.

GREENING YOUR BODY

There's a Green Revolution going on in nutrition. It's due to the recent introduction of high-quality, standardized phytonutrients, or specific nutrient compounds derived from plants. While food is still our best medicine, and there's no substitute for a diverse diet of high-quality fresh and natural foods, specific ingredients have been identified in nature that can be individually studied. After careful characterization and scientific validation, they can be incorporated in reliable, concentrated form to deliver specific benefits.

Among my favorites are the following:

EGCG (Epigallocatechingallate): One of the polyphenol catechins found in green tea, EGCG is known primarily as a cancer-fighter. It also combats inflammation, may counter osteoporosis, and has even been shown to enhance weight loss through its thermogenic properties. Aim for two to four 500 mg capsules daily of EGCG extract, standardized to at least 45 percent concentration.

SGS (sulforaphane glucosinolate): An indole compound derived from cabbage-family vegetables, SGS has been shown to enhance detoxification of harmful environmental pollutants, and to prevent cancer. A potent antioxidant, it can prevent sunburn and reverse serious skin disorders. I like formulas delivering 30 mg sulforaphane glucosinolate per capsule, with a suggested dose of one or two 500 mg capsules daily.

Pycnogenol: A derivative of French maritime pine bark, pycnogenol acts as a strong antioxidant that can protect blood vessels and the brain from free radical damage and inflammation. Lately, research has shown that it can aid recovery from intense exertion. Try to get 85–90 percent pycnogenol, taking one or two 100 mg capsules per day.

Curcumin: A powerful anti-inflammatory derived from the curry spice turmeric, curcumin has been shown to halt the progression of Alzheimer's disease, and may even play a role in staving off cystic fibrosis. High-quality products are standardized to 95 percent curcuminoids, and typical capsules contain 250–400 mg of active ingredient with a recommended daily dose of one capsule twice daily.

GET SOME CULTURE

I wouldn't have said so just a few years back, but probiotics, such as acidophilus, are essential for *everyone* at all life stages. It used to be believed that probiotics were only for people with digestive problems, like gas, bloating, diarrhea, or constipation. But the benefits of probiotics extend way beyond just gastrointestinal health.

Large parts of the immune system reside in the intestines. Normal "cross-talk" between beneficial bacteria in the gut and receptors in the gut wall helps regulate normal immunity. With all the insults to which we subject our GI tract (antibiotics, chlorinated and fluoridated water, antacids, alcohol, toxic food additives), it's no wonder that we experience more immune problems than ever before: frequent infections, autoimmune disorders, even cancer. The aging process compounds the degradation of the healthy flora that populates our guts.

Studies show that people who regularly consume probiotics even have less work absenteeism due to colds and flus!

Look for quality products that incorporate beneficial probiotics like lactobacillus and bifidobacteria. The CFU (colony-forming units) score is a clue to their potency, and ideally should be in the billions.

THE "DUH" STORY OF 21ST-CENTURY NUTRITION

D is for "duh!,", and though I hate to single out just one nutrient as being essential for everyone when so many supplements compete for the distinction, I have to make an exception for vitamin D. There's a cavalcade of conditions in which vitamin D deficiency is implicated:

- Metabolism: Vitamin D has been found to be lower in obese individuals. Supplementation seems to help cells respond better to insulin and blood sugar, as well as help curb fat accumulation around the waist. Some studies have even shown that vitamin D can help lower blood pressure.

- Bones: Researchers believe vitamin D has eclipsed calcium in importance; without adequate vitamin D, the body cannot absorb calcium and utilize it for bone repair. Remarkably, vitamin D prevents fractures in the feeble elderly not just by fortifying bone; it may aid balance and enhance muscle strength to prevent falls.

- Cancer: Studies show that cancer forms clusters in latitudes where vitamin D–generating sunlight is scarce in winter; this may apply, in particular, to cancer of the prostate, breast, and colon, and lymphomas.

- Unexplained body aches: In a recent study of women with "achy body syndrome" not attributable to a specific disease, nearly 90 percent had suboptimal vitamin D levels; restoration of vitamin D levels provided substantial relief to a large majority of pain sufferers.

- Autoimmune disease: Multiple sclerosis is rare in equatorial regions where people get a lot of sunshine; in the wake of promising animal research, the MS Society is currently sponsoring research utilizing high doses of vitamin D to prevent relapses. As in kindred autoimmune diseases, vitamin D helps put the brakes on arthritis. Ultraviolet light exposure and synthetic vitamin D cream help alleviate psoriasis.

- Hyperparathyroidism: It may seem counterintuitive, but adequate levels of vitamin D can actually help bring *down* excess levels of calcium in this condition, which is reaching epidemic proportions, especially among women.

- Immunity: New studies suggest that vitamin D may help combat infections ranging from the infuenza and the common cold to tuberculosis.

- Mood: Why is it we crave those tropical vacations? The key may be vitamin D's depression-alleviating effects.

To top even that, vitamin D may be the ultimate longevity supplement. According to a combined analysis of eighteen clinical trials, intake of modest doses of vitamin D supplements was linked with a 7 percent reduction in overall risk of death.

The list of benefits is so long because vitamin D actually regulates cells, systems, and organs throughout the body.

There's an emerging consensus that very high percentages of the population, especially those in northern latitudes who get little sunlight (which produces vitamin D in the skin), the elderly, and those with darker skin, may be critically deficient in vitamin D, explaining the high prevalence of the above-noted disorders. This has resulted in an urgent call from public health officials to raise the RDA for vitamin D from its current level of 400 IU to 2,000 IU. Certainly 2,000 IU is fine for routine supplementation, but I suggest that everyone ask their doctor for a 25 hydroxy vitamin D blood test to make sure they are in the high-normal range for vitamin D (50 nanograms per milliliter is the level required to gain most of vitamin D's benefits). Many of my patients need more on a selective basis. But high dosing with vitamin D should always be undertaken under the supervision of a health professional because it can accumulate in the body and result in toxicity.

REFINING YOUR NUTRITIONAL PORTFOLIO

That's the core program. To further customize your nutritional portfolio, decide on additional personal health objectives, and add supplements accordingly.

For example, for eye protection, add lutein and zeaxanthin. High-quality eye supplements contain 10 mg of lutein and 2 mg of zeaxanthin per capsule with a recommended daily dose of two capsules per day.

Alternatively, a person concerned with joint health might do well to add glucosamine sulfate or hydrochloride: 1,500 mg; chondroitin: 1200 mg; and MSM: 2–4 grams.

Patients with heart problems would do well to consider coenzyme Q_{10}: 200–500 mg per day; and L-carnitine: 2,000 mg per day.

The possibilities and permutations are literally infinite, since each of us has unique needs. As with investment, enlightened portfolio self-management after proper research and due diligence can be rewarding. But expert help from an experienced and trusted professional is invaluable, particularly if your requirements are complex.

May you reap major health dividends!

11

A Plastic Surgeon's
Secrets to Health

Christine Horner, MD

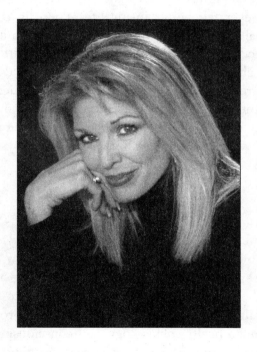

Christine Horner is a board-certified and nationally recognized surgeon, author, professional speaker, and relentless champion for women's health. She spearheaded legislation in the 1990s that made it mandatory for insurance companies to pay for breast reconstruction following mastectomy. She is the author of *Waking the Warrior Goddess: Dr. Christine Horner's Program to Protect Against and Fight Breast Cancer,* winner of the 2006 IPPY award for Best Book in Health, Medicine, and Nutrition. Website: www.drchristinehorner.com

As a plastic surgeon, I specialized in taking care of people seeking to be more youthful. I was able to transform their surface appearance, but did nothing to truly reverse or slow down their aging or to improve their health—I only created an illusion of that. When I was introduced to an ancient system of medicine from India, called ayurveda, and personally experienced its astounding detoxifying, rebalancing, and rejuvenating effects, my approach to and understanding of health, aging, and beauty radically changed. After only forty-eight hours at an ayurvedic clinic, doing a program called *panchakarma* that powerfully detoxifies and rebalances the body, I looked a decade younger and never felt better in my life. There in the mirror, my reflection revealed a markedly younger appearance and a profoundly healthy radiance, which could never be achieved with the knife, or with lasers or chemicals. It was something that could only emanate from a state of remarkable health. That's what my patients were seeking, but with the tools I had as a plastic surgeon, I could never give them what they truly desired. Now I realized that the principles and techniques of ayurveda—a five-thousand-year-old system of medicine—held the secrets to the real fountain of youth.

AYURVEDA

Ayur means "life," and *veda* means "knowledge," so *ayurveda* literally means "the knowledge of life." It's the science of how to live a long, perfectly healthy life by achieving and maintaining a fine state of balance in your physiology. *Ayurveda* teaches how to live life to its fullest potential. It incorporates an in-depth and profound understanding of human health, physiology, and consciousness, and if you follow its advice, you can slow and even reverse aging, and achieve a state of extraordinary and vibrant health beyond what you ever thought possible.

All the techniques and principles in ayurveda boil down to two grand underlying principles. First, *perfect balance brings perfect health*. Ayurveda emphasizes that everything you do or eat—every day—either brings you into balance or throws you out of balance. The trick is to know the difference. If you choose only those foods and activities that bring balance, you can create perfect health. As you might have suspected, the secrets to health and longevity do not lie in a magic pill, plastic surgery, or supplemental hormones. Good health and youthfulness only come as a result of daily health-promoting habits.

Second, *perfect health is achieved through enlivening your inner healing intelligence.* In other words, all health-promoting foods, activities, herbs, and so on, work by making your body stronger and smarter at repairing itself and resisting disease. It's equally important to recognize not only what brings you into balance, but also what throws you out of balance and, therefore, what you should avoid. These are the activities you do or the foods you eat that weaken you and accelerate aging because they violate the natural laws governing your mind/body. Knowing these laws of nature in advance helps to keep you from making the mistakes or adopting the habits that obstruct your inner healing intelligence.

One of my favorite sayings is "You can mop up the water on the floor, but unless you turn off the faucet, you'll never get the floor dry." It doesn't take a rocket scientist to understand that sitting in front of a TV all day, eating junk food, staying up late at night and trying to medicate your stress by smoking and drinking alcohol will not lead to robust health and slowed aging. Whereas, if you eat lots of fresh, organically produced plants—vegetables, fruits, and whole grains—exercise regularly, maintain your ideal weight, get to bed early, practice a stress-reducing technique daily, such as meditation, and supplement your diet with health-promoting substances like antioxidants and omega-3 fatty acids, the chances that you will radiate health, feel great, and slow the aging process are very high. It should be no surprise that a study conducted in London and released in January 2008 found that people who drink moderately, exercise, quit smoking, and eat five servings or more of fruits and vegetables each day live an average of fourteen years longer than people who adopt none of these behaviors.

The principles of ayurveda—which go far beyond the prior basic health advice—are the keys to understanding all the rules that govern your health. When you know the rules and follow them, you receive blessings, avoid catastrophes, and pave the way to the immense pleasure of extraordinary balance, good health, and radiant youthfulness.

MIND/BODY HEALTH BENEFITS
OF TRANSCENDENTAL MEDITATION

Ayurveda emphasizes the experience of higher states of consciousness, which are characterized by an expanded awareness that brings profound balance to the mind/body. Research shows that people who regularly practice techniques that cultivate higher, more expanded states of consciousness—such as transcendental meditation—enjoy so much balance that they are dramatically healthier than the average American. These individuals are found to use the health care system, overall, 50 percent less often and have 87 percent fewer hospital admissions for cardiovascular diseases than their counterparts who do not practice these techniques!

However, the ultimate intention of ayurveda goes far beyond preventing disease. Its goal is to produce robust perfect health for the mind/body and the consciousness. This level of health is of paramount importance because it helps you to achieve higher states of consciousness—and ultimately, enlightenment. Enlightenment is the highest state of human awareness: the ability to see and know the reality of all things and to enjoy mastery over the physical state of being.

More than five hundred studies have been conducted on TM at two-hundred-plus independent institutions and universities in more than thirty different countries. These studies show that the health benefits of experiencing transcendental consciousness daily are nothing short of miraculous. It dramatically reduces stress and anxiety, and promotes good health.

According to the National Institutes of Health (NIH), stress is the cause of, or a major contributing factor in, more than 90 percent of all illnesses, and it also accelerates aging. Because TM radically lowers stress, it also substantially lowers the risk of most diseases and slows aging. The research-proven health benefits of the regular daily practice of TM are numerous, diverse, and impressive. They include lower blood pressure, reversal of coronary artery disease, better mental capacity with improved academic performance, enhanced creativity, and improved verbal and analytical thinking. TM is also associated with less worry, depression, and anxiety; fewer emotional disturbances; and better relationships, job performance, and satisfaction.

TM and Aging

One of the most astonishing findings about the regular practice of TM is that it can *reverse* the aging process. Research shows that individuals who have meditated for more than five years are physiologically about twelve years younger than those who haven't. These conclusions were based on measurements of near-point vision, hearing, and systolic (the higher number) blood pressure—all of which predictably worsen with age.

As you age, the levels of hormones in your body also change. For example, you produce much less of the hormone dehydroepiandosterone sulfate (DHEA)—the most abundant hormone found in young adults. DHEA has many positive effects on your body, one of which is building lean muscle mass. After your mid-thirties, you begin to lose lean muscle mass, and declining DHEA levels are thought be largely responsible for this phenomenon. Research shows that you can slow down the rate at which DHEA levels fall and stay physiologically younger by exercising and practicing TM. In general, the level of DHEA in meditators is the same as that normally found in individuals five to ten years younger.

For women, keeping DHEA levels higher is important for two additional reasons: DHEA is protective against both breast cancer and osteoporosis. Research shows that women who have high DHEA levels have a lower risk of both of these diseases.

OTHER STRESS-REDUCING TECHNIQUES

Although TM has been found to be the most effective form of meditation, other types of meditation can be beneficial, too. Be aware, however, that research shows that certain types of meditation using concentration techniques may actually increase anxiety, so I would avoid them. If you cannot arrange to learn TM, there are other good stress-reducing and health-promoting practices, such as yoga or the breathing technique called *pranayama*, which can provide you with excellent health benefits. Don't forget that daily exercise is also a stress-buster.

AN ANCIENT AYURVEDIC ANTI-AGING FORMULA

Amrit Kalash was originally designed, thousands of years ago, as an anti-aging formula. Ayurveda considers *Amrit Kalash* to be something called a *rasayana*. The word *rasayana* is from the Sanskrit language; it means "that which negates old age and disease." Research has shown that *Amrit Kalash* can indeed slow the aging process because it's such a powerful antioxidant. Aging is accelerated by oxygen-free radicals, and antioxidants neutralize them.

Dr. Yukie Niwa, a Japanese researcher, studied more than five hundred different antioxidants over a period of thirty years. He found that the most powerful and effective antioxidant of all those tested is an ancient ayurvedic herbal preparation called *Amrit Kalash*. Research shows that the antioxidant capabilities of *Amrit Kalash* are at least 25,000 times more powerful than those of vitamins C and E. This astounding ambrosia is composed of forty-four different herbs and fruits that seem to work synergistically, enhancing the natural strength of one another's antioxidants.

Due to its extraordinary antioxidants (and countless other health-protecting and wellness-enhancing nutrients), *Amrit Kalash* also defends against a variety of chronic disorders, including cancer, in significant ways. For instance, it prevents tumors from starting, slows down tumor growth, and even shrinks tumors.

Research shows that *Amrit Kalash* may actually *reverse* aging. In a double-blind, placebo-controlled study, patients who received *Amrit Kalash* improved significantly on an age-related alertness task. Performance of this task is known to highly correlate with age. The older you are, the worse you normally do on this test. This study showed that *Amrit Kalash* could enhance the capacity for attention and alertness that predictably declines with age.

THE QUANTUM APPROACH
TO HEALTH AND LONGEVITY

The principles of ayurveda are actually based on quantum physics. Quantum physics tells us that at the most basic level of life, everything in the Universe is the same, connected, and thought to be made of vibrating strings—physicists call it Superstring Theory. These ing strings cause everything to have a frequency. Scientists have actually measured the frequencies emitted by healthy cells and various organs and tissues in the human body. The frequency of unhealthy cells can be changed to a healthy frequency through a variety of different modalities that use frequency. For example, light, sound, vibration, and certain machines and devices that produce frequency have all been shown to have profound effects on health. Using frequency as medicine is like watering the roots of a tree—it affects everything in the living organism. For example, Transcendental Meditation is thought to work through frequency and that it why it has been shown to improve all aspects of our health: mental, physical, emotional, and spiritual.

I also want to mention an extraordinary "quantum" device that I was first introduced to about a year ago—a cozy, relaxing chamber that uses light, sound, frequency, and vibration to balance and detoxify the body—with results that have been nothing short of miraculous for a variety of ailments. Invented by Barry McNew in Cottonwood, Arizona, the Life Vessel is a simple, safe, and effective method to restore optimum health—so effective that it was recently certified by the FDA. Administered in four one-hour sessions over the course of three days, it is a wonderful way to help detoxify your body, reduce stress, and maintain excellent health. Currently there are four Life Vessel Centers in the United States: in Cottonwood, Arizona; Santa Fe, New Mexico; Tulsa, Oklahoma; and Pittsburgh, Pennsylvania. Several more locations are scheduled to open soon. For more information, go to www.lifevesselsantafe.com

NO MAGIC BULLET

As much as we might wish it, there are no magic bullets, surgery, pills, or supplemental hormones that will create good health, longevity, and youthfulness. These qualities only come from daily health-promoting habits. If you want to get the full joy out of life—and who doesn't?—good health is the key. That requires education, commitment, and action. It doesn't have to be difficult or boring. Rather, it can be exciting and fun. I approach it as an adventure: How good can I feel and look? So now, how good can *you* feel and look?

12

Health and Longevity
for Women

Tori Hudson, ND

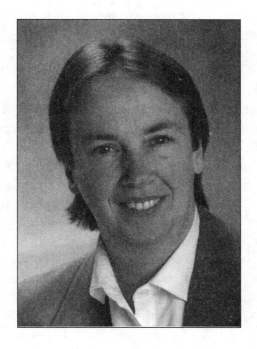

Tori Hudson is one of the foremost experts on women's health issues.
She is the director of A Woman's Time, a clinic in Portland, Oregon, and
the author of the *Women's Encyclopedia of Natural Medicine*. Address:
2067 NW Lovejoy, Portland, OR 97209. Tel: 503-222-2322. Websites:
www.Awomanstime.com and www.Torihudson.com

n thinking about healthy aging, I can't help but think about the beginning, the fountain from which one springs, so to speak. In my case, I had a fortunate youth in so many ways—growing up in a small town on the Oregon Coast, living in view of the bay and next to an old-growth Douglas fir forest, a childhood of athletics, a mother who insisted I eat an apple a day, and parents who made certain I had a good education and lots of opportunities. When asked to share my secrets of health and longevity from the fountain of youth, I'm thinking it's as much about these influences on my young growing body, mind, and spirit, as it is about habits and activities in my adult life.

I was fortunate to gain lifelong health benefits from growing up in the coastal fog belt with no possibility of long-term sun damage to my skin, that one apple a day, seasonal fruit and vegetables always available in the refrigerator, and regular fresh ocean fish. This was in an era when Mom was home cooking meals of real food, rather than prepackaged quasi-food. I also had two to four hours a day of rigorous exercise in my athletic training from the age of seven on, teachers who saw who I was, opportunities to evolve my life in a purposeful way, and a life full of rivers and beaches, and forests. I wish these things and more for all of us. They provide a fundamentally great foundation for good long-term habits, good health, and a vital life. I'm grateful every day for how these experiences influenced my own life and my professional life as a physician.

But even if we didn't have a great start in life, it's not too late to make a big impact on our quality of life now, and our future. In my clinical practice working with women and their health issues, that's what I try to do: Identify and treat current issues or diseases, and prevent or reduce the risk of future problems. For women, the current problems range from simple infections to more complex hormonal problems, mood disorders, chronic serious degenerative diseases, and serious life-threatening diseases. Cardiovascular disease, osteoporosis, breast cancer, diabetes, and osteoarthritis are the big diseases we think about for women. But most of us have mild to severe problems along the path of life. Those need relief, because whether they are short term or, especially, if they are regularly recurring, they can wear us down. Think how insomnia can create fatigue and depression, or how recurring migraine pain not only creates suffering, but can lead to a smaller, severely circumscribed life because the sufferer just doesn't feel like going out. Even simple digestive problems can alter our social and work life. My main point is this: Let's not get overly caught up in the future and what we can do to prevent significant diseases; rather, let's focus on what can we do now to feel better today.

EATING HABITS

In thinking about secrets of health and longevity, I can't help but notice how individual it is. What's going to be an optimal diet for one woman is not necessarily right for others. In my clinical practice, I'm mindful of and attentive to research on various foods, vitamins, minerals, herbs, hormones, and lifestyle habits on prevention and treatment of chronic degenerative diseases. We can find all kinds of research, for example, on how green tea or a low-fat diet can reduce the risk of certain cancers. We can look to the effect of a high-fiber diet on reducing the risk of cardiovascular disease. Diets high in antioxidants and flavonoids slow oxidative damage and reduce inflammation in all kinds of cells and tissues and body systems. We can review the scientific findings on Mediterranean diets in terms of reducing the risk and damage of cardiovascular disease, metabolic syndrome, and diabetes. And what about those fish oils? The list is long in its benefits for our immune system and joints; in reducing inflammation, brain aging, heart disease; and promoting healthy eyes.

There are many diets and nutritional specifics that we can look to for their significant effects on our health. In my opinion, it comes down to both basic themes and specifics.

The basic themes:

- Avoid overeating
- Strive for moderation and balance
- Eat "slow food" and local foods

The specifics:

- Adopt a diet dominated by "healthy fats," vegetables and fruits, whole grains, nuts and seeds, legumes, fish, and modest amounts of meat and dairy products

- Minimize consumption of or avoid sugar, white-flour products, saturated fats, "bad fats," deep-fried, highly processed, and fast greasy foods

A healthy approach to weight loss for women who are overweight is one of the more significant strategies I can offer for long-term health benefits. The goal is to come up with a plan that each individual will follow—one that is safe, effective, and sustainable for a long-term lifestyle. I'm an advocate of Mediterranean-style diets for many. But, as I said earlier, I have to understand and create an individual approach that takes into account the specifics of each woman's physiology and current health problems, her tastes, her vulnerabilities, her psychological relationship with food, and her obstacles to success. Women lose weight differently and at different rates than men, especially for women in their forties to sixties. It's tougher at that age—plain and simple. Working closely with a practitioner and, for many, a therapist and/or personal health coach, is the team approach that is needed to achieve sustained success. Losing weight takes education/information, time, commitment, personal struggle, and patience. The rewards are immense and lifelong, and life will be longer.

EXERCISE

Yes, we have to talk about this. But, most important, we have to do it. There's no getting around exercise for good health and longevity. This is the single most important habit for long-term health. I would assert that regular exercise offers more health benefits than any single diet, vitamin, mineral, herb, or drug. The therapeutic benefits of exercise are phenomenal: Research has shown that exercise treats and/or prevents depression, anxiety, insomnia, PMS, breast cancer, arthritis, hypertension, dangerously high cholesterol levels, cardiovascular disease of all kinds, osteoporosis, diabetes, obesity and its deleterious consequences, and various types of cancers.

Exercise guidelines vary with the scientific study and the goal you are trying to accomplish, but, mostly, more is better. For perimenopausal and menopausal women, especially those who want to lose weight, it likely takes sixty to ninety minutes per day of aerobic exercise. WOW!!! A hard pill to swallow, but one that does indeed work. For added benefits, twenty minutes of strength training just twice a week—but preferably three times a week—will enhance the success of weight loss. To reduce the risks of cardiovascular disease, it's not necessary to be as rigorous and thirty minutes a minimum of four days a week are effective, but even better results are achieved with daily aerobic exercise. We don't have to get fancy with our aerobics— walking works, and it's free and doable any place, any time. If you've got bad knees or other physical limitations, then we find what is appropriate—stationary bike? rowing machine? swimming?

An adult life of healthy whole foods, regular exercise, selected supplements, connecting with the beauty and spirit of mother nature, a spiritual connection with self and surrounding oneself with a community of people who share similar values seems like a formula for optimal living and one that supports optimal aging.

SUPPLEMENTS

There are so many possibilities to consider for disease treatment and prevention in women. Where I would start is what is going on now that needs treatment, and then what are the conditions/diseases that my patient is at increased risk for. Fortunately, we get a lot of bang for our buck with some supplements because they have effects on multiple systems. Fish oils, green tea, vitamin D, flavonoids, and curcumin are standouts for me. It's interesting to me that these are nutrients that are reflected in the diets and lifestyle of cultures known for their health. Fish oils are associated with many health benefits for the eyes (forestalling macular degeneration), the heart (staving off stroke, atherosclerosis, heart attacks), the immune system (decreased inflammation and improved immune responses), as well as alleviating chronic pain, diabetes, brain disorders (depression and other mood disorders, attention deficit disorder, autism, learning skills, cognitive decline), and enhancing maternal and fetal health.

Green tea is associated with reducing the risk of cardiovascular disease, plus breast and ovarian cancer; inhibiting the human papilloma virus and treating cervical dysplasia; treating polycystic ovarian syndrome; and increasing weight loss.

Those of us with higher vitamin D levels circulating in our blood or those of us who live in sunnier latitudes have lower rates of cardiovascular disease, autoimmune diseases, breast and ovarian cancer, and depression. Supplementing with vitamin D also slows bone loss and reduces the risk of fractures, and taking vitamin D supplements will achieve the same results as getting the vitamin from sunshine.

Flavonoids are a group of plant pigments that are mostly responsible for the bright colors of our fruits, vegetables, and flowers. Flavonoids are found in supplements of different sizes and shapes: proanthocyanidins (PCO from grape seed and pine bark), quercetin, citrus bioflavonoids, and green tea polyphenols. Collectively, flavonoids are known as nature's "biological response modifiers," meaning they can modify the body's reaction to many compounds, including allergens, viruses, and carcinogens. In essence, they have anti-inflammatory, anti-allergenic, antiviral, and anticarcinogenic properties, in addiction to acting as powerful antioxidants, providing protection against oxidative and free radical damage.

Turmeric, or its curcumin extract, is derived from the ginger family. Turmeric/curcumin is the major ingredient in curry powder and is used extensively in Chinese, Indonesian, and Indian cooking and systems of medicine. The pharmacological effects of curcumin are many: It is been shown to be an effective antioxidant, anti-inflammatory, anticarcinogenic, and antimicrobial agent. In addition, it has beneficial effects on the liver, and the cardiovascular and digestive systems. Curcumin is used in the prevention and adjuvant treatment of cancers, as well as in lowering cholesterol levels, inhibiting blood clots, treating hepatitis/irritable bowel syndrome/gallstones/arthritis, and curbing the growth of organisms that cause common infections. Curcumin is one of the most common herbs I prescribe for my patients, given its wide and potent range of effects.

THE PERSONAL

I know there are many prominent researchers, healers, and clinicians who can speak much more articulately than I about the power of thought or prayer or meditation or ceremony on health and healing.

In my clinical practice and work with women, I try to awaken in them an awareness of a deeper connection with their lives, the people in their lives, a spiritual relationship with some force, and the deeper process of healing. I try to listen for what that might be for them and then identify resources they can access to evolve in this way. I deeply respect all the possible individual ways that might look in a particular woman's life, so I have no specific agenda here other than to try to inspire or increase the rigorousness of the search and the connection. As part of this process, I believe that connecting with nature is a powerful force that can be incorporated into anyone's belief system. In naturopathic medicine, we have a principle called the healing power of nature or the *vis medicatrix naturae*, which means that the body has the inherent ability to establish, maintain, and restore health. My role, as physician, is to facilitate and augment this process with the aid of natural, nontoxic therapies; to act to identify and remove obstacles to health and recovery; and to support the creation of a healthy internal and external environment. But, literally, there is a healing power of nature—the healing force of being in, being with, experiencing the beauty of, the balance within, and the powers of mother nature.

SUMMARY

Some profound secrets or advice or ways of life have been shared with me by other teachers. Traditional Seventh-day Adventists talk about the seven natural remedies: Nutrition, Exercise, Water, Sunshine, Temperance, Air, and Trust in Divine Power. They call it NEW-START. The Navajo have a spiritual basis for their lives, to "walk in beauty," and I have treasured the meaning of this on every level. The Dalai Lama has a message of kindness. And a way of life I have gleaned from living and watching the lives of others is that of generosity.

I will continue to recommend my not-so-secret secrets of vitality to the women I work with: healthy diets, regular exercise, selected supplements, and well-being in one's personal and spiritual life, but I think it may come down to each of us living our lives as though we have everything to do with the outcome, while also praying and trusting that some higher power/s has everything to do with it.

13

Healthy Relationships and Longevity

Ron Hunninghake, MD

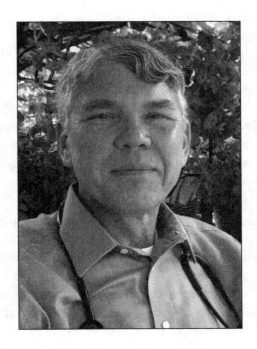

Ron Hunninghake is chief medical officer at the Center for the Improvement of Human Functioning in Wichita, Kansas, the largest nonprofit nutritional medicine center in the United States. He is the coauthor (with Jack Challem) of *Stop Prediabetes*. Address: 3100 N. Hillside Ave, Wichita, KS 67219. Tel: 316-682-3100. E-mail: bcri@brightspot.org. Website: www.brightspot.org

Friendship is a plant we must often water.
—Shalom Aleichem

Most people intuitively know that the quality of their important relationships impacts their health. Who hasn't heard that famous soap opera line, delivered by the maligned spouse to his or her unfaithful, ungrateful, or critical spouse: "I'm sick and tired of you."

Researchers at UCLA have scientifically confirmed this *relationship* relationship—namely that women in happy marriages recover more quickly from workday stress than women in unhappy relationships. Other studies have found that married men live longer and recover faster from illness than single men. This phenomenon is true for women too, if their marriages are happy. The research begs an important question: Just what is a "happy" marriage? What makes one relationship good and another bad?

Of course, most of us know when we feel happy. We can pick out a strong relationship when we are in one. Our so-called emotional intelligence "knows" what a good relationship is and most of us certainly prefer a good one over a bad one. We even *know* that good ones are better for our health than bad ones. It really doesn't take scientific research to confirm this emotional truism.

Why, then, do so many people have so much trouble with relationships? Are we purposefully choosing to remain in bad relationships? Do we want to be sick? Or is it that we just haven't learned *how* to cultivate a healthy relationship?

The answer is surprising: We *do* know how to cultivate healthy relationships! Almost all of us do it, even as kids. But running parallel to this fundamental knowledge is a set of insidious cultural assumptions that often doom our efforts to live in healthy relationships.

Okay. It is possible that there are people reading this piece who have *never* had a friend, and tragically know nothing about friendship. It is possible, but unlikely. Even evil people seek the company of other evil people.

Quintus Ennius succinctly stated that "Life is nothing without friendship." Your experience in friendships is the touchstone that will reveal the essence of a healthy relationship. But not every human relationship is a friendship. Or is it?

Let's look at the major types of relationships all of us experience, and consider the degree of choice that we are given in each category:

- Friend–Friend (always a choice)
- Husband–Wife (initially a choice)
- Parent–Child (not a choice)
- Teacher–Student (not much of a choice)
- Boss–Employee (not much of a choice)
- Doctor–Patient (not much of a choice)

Not everyone reading this essay will have experienced all these relationship categories. I'm going to assume, for the sake of argument, that all my readers have experienced friendship. This leads to a basic question: Are friendships less problematic (and more happy) than other relationships? If you think so, why?

FRIENDSHIPS VERSUS RELATIONSHIPS

	Freely Chosen?	Problematic?
Friendships	Yes	Rarely
Relationships	Often not	Commonly

The above table asserts that true friendships are freely chosen and rarely problematic. Granted, any relationship—even a friendship—can become problematic, but only when the principle of free choice is violated. How does this element of free choice enter into relationship dynamics?

Healthy relationships are built on the assumption of the intrinsic freedom of choice. Unhealthy relationships are built on the assumption of *external control*—a term coined by psychiatrist Dr. William Glasser in his 1998 book, *Choice Theory*. What does Dr. Glasser mean by external control?

External control is a psychological assumption that holds that you can and somehow deserve to control those you are in important relationships with (except friends!). The depth of this assumption commonly obscures our awareness of it. If you find yourself criticizing, blaming, complaining, nagging, threatening, punishing, and/or bribing someone you are in a relationship with in order to control his or her behavior, then external control is your hidden assumption made manifest.

External control violates our intrinsic need to be free. Do you feel nourished when you are with a controlling person? Do you even want to be with him? Or are you trapped by the external circumstances of that particular relationship (child, spouse, boss, insurance doctor, etc.)?

External control is often dictated by the contractual nature of many of our important relationships. Marriage, in the legal sense, is a contract. Your job is often dictated by a contract. Doctor-patient relationships may be contractual through an insurance program. Many consider responsible parenting an unwritten contract. Contracts necessarily restrict freedom of choice by binding us to specific agreements. When we break those agreements, there are consequences.

But even in a contract, we were free to enter into it. The spirit of any good contract is grounded in a mutual benefit to both parties. Good contracts are based on the following:

- Listening
- Supporting
- Encouraging
- Respecting

- Trusting
- Accepting
- Always negotiating disagreements

These are the seven caring habits that Glasser feels are so essential to healthy relationships—even legal ones! In essence, the best contracts are made between friends.

I'll bet you are saying to yourself: "I already know all this!" If you do, then you know the secret of healthy relationships. If your life is peppered with broken, grief-stricken relationships, then maybe there's more you need to learn.

Glasser sums it all up with this question: "How can I figure out how to be free to live my life the way I want to live it and still get along well with the people I need?" Each of us must strive to achieve that connectedness with others in a way that preserves our individual freedom while simultaneously meeting our basic needs to belong and be cared for, to be respected and listened to, to have fun, and to be free to choose.

A tall order you say. How is it possible? Do we have to attend some kind of intensive relationship seminar to learn how to do it? No. We merely have to remember what it is to be a friend.

A friend listens. A friend supports. A friend encourages. A friend is trustworthy. A friend respects. A friend accepts. A friend is always willing to negotiate disagreements. A friend is, well, a friend.

When friendship becomes the basic assumption of all our important relationships, then the spirit of connectedness is alive and well. The relationship can breathe. Need fulfillment, mutual benefits, and responsibility through service become the life and soul of those relationships.

Choice theory asks us to responsibly create and maintain healthy relationships. External control psychology, by contrast, is based on a strange but common line of thought:

- I am not responsible for the way I feel.

- Other people, unhappy events, or abnormal brain chemistry cause my pain.

- My choices are not the cause of my misery.

- To feel better:
  - I will punish the people who are doing wrong, so that they will do what I say is right;
  - I will then reward them, so that they will keep doing what I want them to do.

In essence, external control uses the blame game as a means to meet our basic needs. Blame justifies control. Control does meet our need to be listened to, but at the expense of our need to be loved and to belong. And control is no fun. The great lessons of history tell us that control never lasts. Our human need for freedom is too great.

So why do we do it? Why do we perpetuate unhealthy relationships through the application of external control? We do it because it seems to work in the short term. When you yell, threaten, criticize, blame, punish, and bribe, you get "results." People will respond and change their behavior—temporarily. But the life of the relationship will begin to die a little bit. The connectedness will erode. Agreements will begin to be broken. Usually, it is only a matter of time before that relationship will either quietly or dramatically end.

Do we learn? Unfortunately, 99 percent of humankind will choose these behaviors over and over. Rarely do we stop to think how much misery these behaviors cause us. This psychology of coercion destroys happiness, health, marriages, families, and quality work. It is often the root cause of the violence, crime, drug abuse, illness, and unloving sex so pervasive in our society.

What small bit of wisdom do I have to contribute to this mess? Just this little aphorism: "The smart bird does not poop in its own nest."

We live in our important relationships. All our basic needs as humans are met in these relationships. They deserve to be handled with care. Pay attention to the feelings of others as if they were your own. Take time to listen and sort things out. Don't speak impulsively. Spend time together. Have some fun. Cultivate, cultivate, cultivate. Healthy relationships, like friendships, don't just happen: They are cultivated!

Choice theory states that the only person I can control is myself. Since controlling the other is often counterproductive, why not ask "What can *I* do to improve my relationships?" Ironically, others almost always change as we stop trying to externally control them and begin paying attention to their basic human needs. Why not ask, "What can I do to help my _____ satisfy his or her basic needs?"

In summary, healthy relationships are good for your health. Friendship is the universal basis of healthy relationships. We can cultivate healthy relationships ("connectedness") by listening, supporting, encouraging, respecting, trusting, accepting, and always negotiating disagreements. These habits of caring are much more effective at building quality relationships than the destructive habits of criticizing, blaming, complaining, nagging, threatening, punishing, bribing (or rewarding in order to control).

Friendship is a choice you make. In order to have good friendships and healthy relationships, be a good friend first. You'll increase your chances of greater happiness, and you'll probably live longer, too!

14

My Quest
for the Fountain

Beatrice Trum Hunter, MA

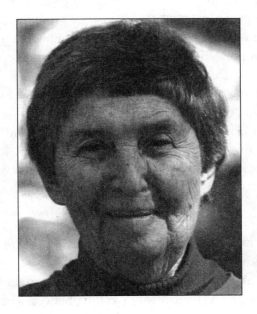

Beatrice Trum Hunter, a pioneering consumer health writer, has focused her long career on food and environmental issues. She is the author of *Food and Your Health, The Natural Foods Cookbook, Gardening Without Poisons,* and many other books. She has also served as the food editor of *Consumers' Research Magazine.* Address: Hillsboro, NH.

People have been drawn to fountains because fountains have represented a source of knowledge, health, the life force, and, for Ponce de León and others, a restoration of youthfulness. In the thirteenth century, a French metalsmith built a silver fountain for the Mongol prince, Mangu Khan, in the main square of Karakoram. The fountain had four spouts, which dispensed, respectively, koumiss (mare's milk), wine, mead, and rice wine. Were the offerings of this early vending machine, from fermented milk, fruit, honey, and grain, an attempt to bestow health and longevity? Perhaps.

My own quest for knowledge about food, nutrition, and health has centered mainly around books. They have served as the source of my understanding about the vital role played by good foods and nutrition as they relate to good health. Indeed, books continue to be important in my ever-evolving understanding of various aspects of nutrition. Books have influenced the direction of my life.

I was raised in a household where white bread and foods made with copious amounts of sugar and Crisco predominated. There were few vegetables and fruits. Up to my college years, my body reflected this dreadful diet. Repeatedly, I developed dental caries. I suffered from acne, lusterless hair, frequent headaches, and a low level of energy.

THE EPIPHANY

A muckraking book changed my life. Titled *100,000,000 Guinea Pigs: Dangers in Everyday Foods, Drugs, and Cosmetics* and coauthored by Arthur Kallet and F. J. Schlink from the independent organization Consumers' Research, Inc., this book documented what was happening to the American public—a population of 100 million at the time. The book related case studies in the files of Consumers' Research, which demonstrated how poorly the public was protected against the dangers in the marketplace. The authors dared to reveal brand names of offending products, a practice that made publishers leery of accepting the work for fear of a libel suit. Ultimately, a courageous publisher, Vanguard Press, published the book in 1933. The book became a best-seller.

The book shocked me. I began to take charge of my food choices and changed my eating habits. I limited sugar-laden foods and drinks, and shunned frankfurters and lunch meats. I began to eat many more vegetables and fruits, and added some that previously had been unfamiliar to me. I learned to enjoy the taste and texture of whole-grain porridges and breads. Before long, I began to notice changes in myself. My skin was clearer, my hair shone, the headaches disappeared, and I had more energy. The damage already inflicted on my teeth could not be reversed, but I no longer developed new cavities. I was convinced that my dietary changes were responsible for these health improvements. I was eager to learn more about foods, nutrition, and health.

THE QUEST BEGINS

Being an avid reader, I found many books on food, nutrition, and health. I was confused. Statements and ideas expressed by some authors seemed contradictory. Others seemed to offer unsound, even dangerous advice. I felt that basic nutritional concepts needed to be sound and well tested by human experience.

I found the answers in another book that shaped my ideas profoundly. It was *Nutrition and Physical Degeneration* by Weston A. Price, DDS (1945). Dr. Price described the good health maintained by people in various parts of the world who followed traditional diets. Unfortunately, their health would deteriorate rapidly once they switched to a diet of industrialized foods. Although Dr. Price's original plan was to study dental health, he soon realized that the entire body, mind, and spirit were affected by nutrition. Intelligence, physical endurance, mental outlook, ease of childbirth, lack of degenerative diseases that plague developed countries, and other factors, were all related to good nutrition. Price's findings had an important message for us: Eat basic foods, as fresh as possible, produced on fertile, poison-free soil.

My early readings were simple. As I progressed, the subjects seemed to broaden out to include connections that were unanticipated. For example, the Kallet and Schlink book had been written before the DDT era, but the authors had described the use of lead arsenate sprays in apple orchards. The subject of pesticides needed to be included in any quest for good nutrition. Kallet and Schlink touched on changes in agricultural practices that decreased the nutritional value of foods. This was another aspect to examine. The book discussed the beginnings of the food revolution, with the accelerated pace of production of highly processed, factory-prepared food products, accompanied by the prolific use of chemical additives, such as sulfiting agents and food dyes.

The Kallet and Schlink book stimulated me to search for earlier works on food adulteration, including Frederick Accum's *Death in the Pot* (circa 1830), Upton Sinclair's *The Jungle* (1906), Dr. Harvey W. Wiley's *The History of a Crime against a Food Law* (1929), as well as numerous FDA recalls and U.S. General Accounting Office reports on the subject. It was important for me to gain a historical perspective.

Similarly, there were enlightening follow-ups in the Kallet and Schlink tradition. Notable ones were Dr. Ross Hume Hall's *Food for Nought* (1974), Eric Schlosser's *Fast Food Nation: The Dark Side of the All-American Meal* (2001), and Marion Nestle's *Food Politics* (2002).

After reading Dr. Price's book, I searched for earlier writings in support of his findings. Among them were the works of Drs. Robert McCarrison, H. P. Pickerell, Francis M. Pottenger Jr., John Myers, G. T. Wrench, George V. Mann, Otto Schaeffer, and Lady Eve Balfour. In more recent years, Price's findings have been confirmed by Drs. Michael Crawford, S. Boyd Eaton, Melvin Konner, Joseph D. Beasley, and Melvin Page, among others.

Fortunately, even in my rural location, my library was helpful in obtaining requested books through the interlibrary loan system. For more recently published books, the Mildred Hatch Free Lending Library was invaluable. Mildred Hatch and her husband, Ira Hatch, ran a mail-order business of natural foods from their modest home in Middlebury, Vermont, during the 1940s and 1950s. They filled orders everywhere for staples, such as dried beans, nuts, seeds, grains, dried fruits, and nutritional yeast. This business, unique at the time, supported the free lending library. Books could be borrowed for a time, with no charge other than postage. Although there was no obligation to purchase the books, they were available for sale to those who wished to purchase them. This free library service was a wonderful opportunity for individuals like me to slake a thirst for knowledge.

My readings extended to government publications as well as scientific and medical journals. As I read, many questions arose. Often, I would request reprints of papers. I found that many authors were happy to learn that there were individuals out there who actually read their writings. They were eager to discuss their findings, and sometimes provided additional articles than those I had requested to extend my understanding. As a result, I began to acquire mentors in various fields. Two of them influenced my thinking to a large extent.

TWO MENTORS

Theron G. Randolph, MD, was one of my most treasured mentors. Our interests overlapped in the areas of foods, food additives, and pesticides. However, Randolph did pioneering work that encompassed far more. He broke new ground in understanding the impact of the total environment on human health. His seminal book, *Human Ecology and Susceptibility to the Chemical Environment* (1962) expanded my own understanding. I cherished him as a patient mentor who encouraged my own efforts. Our friendship endured for five decades until his death.

F. J. Schlink not only became one of my great mentors, but also became my publisher, my sharp-eyed editor, and my cherished friend until his death at the age of 103. Several decades after having read *100,000,000 Guinea Pigs*, I wrote a very belated note of thanks to Mr. Schlink and told him about the profound influence the book had had on my life. When I wrote to him, he was president of Consumers' Research, Inc. and publisher of its monthly publication, *Consumers' Research* magazine. He had established the organization in 1928, and its publications were well respected for their truthfulness and reliability. The organization was fiercely independent and never accepted any funding either from industry or government. It was totally unbiased. Schlink responded to my note, and soon we began a lively exchange of letters and clippings with notes added in the margins, or sections underscored. This correspondence continued for many years. At some point, Schlink asked if I would consider writing an occasional piece for the magazine. At first, he suggested topics for me to develop. Later, he accepted my own suggestions. After some time, I wrote the food and nutrition section for the magazine's *Annual.* Then, my work expanded to a monthly column and feature articles, as well as answering readers' questions about food and nutrition. Ultimately, I served as food editor for twenty years, until the demise of *Consumers' Research* in 2004.

THE QUEST EXPANDS

Nutrition is an evolving science. At the time of early pioneers, such as Drs. Wilbur O. Atwater (working in the nineteenth century) and Elmer V. McCollum (active in the early twentieth century), the basic nutrients had been identified. Gradually, the importance of trace elements became recognized. Tiny in size, they exert profound effects nevertheless. The pioneering work of Drs. Firman Bear, William Albrecht, André Voisin, Karl Schutte, and Henry A. Schroeder added to my expanding understanding of nutrition. Then, along came the discovery of a whole new set of substances—phytochemicals in foods —which expanded the complexities. What next? Be prepared for the discovery of additional substances, as yet unknown and unidentified, but important for our ever-expanding nutritional understanding. If anything, the subject is open-ended, and the searcher constantly needs to be ready to readjust, reevaluate, incorporate insights from new findings, and modify or even reject former ideas. This pattern is frustrating and confusing, yet challenging and exhilarating!

MY CONCLUSIONS—AT LEAST FOR THE PRESENT

After a lifetime spent searching for valid information about foods, nutrition, and health, what are my conclusions? Actually, they are quite simple, and easy to understand. To follow them, however, is more difficult. Unless you are willing to be unorthodox in your food selections by shunning the typical industrialized diet, you will find obstacles to overcome. Like Odysseus, you will need to stop your ears (and cover your eyes) against the sirens' calls of food product advertisements.

What should you eat? Choose basic foods that were familiar to your forebears, prior to the industrialization of food. These basic foods are eggs, poultry, muscle and organ meats, marrow bones, finfish and shellfish, vegetables, legumes, fruits, nuts, and seeds. If you can tolerate them, consume dairy products. Also, if you can tolerate them, eat whole grains. Both dairy products and grains have entered the human experience relatively recently, with the establishment of stable agriculture only some ten thousand to twenty thousand years ago. This is a short period for adaptation by the human digestive tract. As a result, lactose intolerance, milk allergy, and gluten intolerance may be experienced by some individuals.

SOME DOS AND DON'TS

Eat eggs as frequently as you wish. Eggs are a nutrient-dense, quality-protein, balanced food. Unfortunately, they have been maligned due to misguided concerns about cholesterol. Cooking eggs gently with moist heat is best. Poaching, shirring, coddling, or soft boiling are good methods. The white should be opaque. Hard frying is undesirable. Do not eat raw or undercooked eggs, as in Caesar salad, some homemade eggnog recipes, or meringues. Refrigerate eggs in their original cardboard container, and do not transfer them to the door wells in refrigerators. If the eggs are sold in plastic containers, save a formerly used cardboard container and transfer the eggs to it, since plastic molecules tend to migrate into adjacent foods. Eggs can be stored in the refrigerator for several weeks. They will still be safe to eat, but over time, there will be a gradual decline in nutrients and flavor. Do not purchase cracked eggs or "leakers." Whenever possible, buy eggs from hens raised organically or biodynamically. There is no difference in white- or brown-shelled eggs, nor between small and large eggs. All shell eggs are nourishing. Shun egg substitutes.

Select quality poultry as you select quality eggs. The birds should be free-range. Seek those with the USDA organic seal. If available, buy locally raised birds that are fresh, and have not been frozen previously. Do not attempt to cook a whole bird in a microwave oven. This appliance may cook unevenly, and is unsuitable for whole chickens, turkeys, or meat roasts. Undercooked portions in the bird's interior may contain viable pathogens. Use a traditional oven or a convection oven to cook whole birds or roasts. Also, it is best to cook stuffing separately, for the same reason. If you have an opportunity to vary your poultry intake, eat squab, quail, turkey, duck, or goose, in addition to chicken. If you have a chance, try wildfowl, too. This practice widens your food base, and fulfills the advice to eat as wide a variety of foods as possible.

Fish is nourishing, but some types are more desirable than others. Fatty fishes, such as salmon, mackerel, and herring, contain the beneficial omega-3 fatty acids. Select wild fish whenever possible. For example, wild salmon has far more omega-3 fatty acids (and flavor) than farmed salmon; other fishes likely to be farmed include catfish, trout, tilapia, and shrimp. Certain fish species have high mercury levels. These include swordfish, fresh tuna, and tilefish. Limit or avoid eating them. Although freshly caught fish is desirable, fast-frozen fish from relatively unpolluted areas (for example, Iceland) may be a better choice than fresh fish from polluted areas. Cook all fish thoroughly. Avoid eating raw or undercooked fish, such as oysters, clams, or herring, or dishes like sushi, ceviche, or sashimi. Frequently, such fish contain live bacteria, viruses, or parasites. Everyone is at risk, and people with liver disease or weakened immune systems are at increased risk.

Include organ meats, such as liver, as well as muscle meats, in your food choices. Use marrow bones to make broth or stock, the basis of soups and stews. Eat the marrow. Cook meat thoroughly. Moist heat used for soups and stews is best. Heavily broiled, charbroiled, or grilled meats are unhealthy. Discard any burnt sections of meat.

Despite bad press, animal fats are good, especially if they are from grass-grazed animals. Used in moderation, butter is good. So are chicken, duck, and goose fats. Both butter and coconut oil are good for cooking. Good-quality olive oil and flaxseed oil are good for salad dressings. Other good sources of oil are found in avocado, nuts, seeds, and olives. Gentle sautéeing is preferable to pan-frying or deep-fat frying. Throw out the margarine and other hydrogenated oils and fats. Do not use polyunsaturated oils: They are refined and frequently rancid because they are unstable.

Eat fruits, berries, melons, and all vegetables available. Eat fruits and vegetables rather than drinking their juices. Choose an orange over orange juice; a tomato over tomato juice.

Consume nuts and seeds liberally. They are nutrient-dense. Embrace the age-old tradition of using lacto-fermented foods, such as raw sauerkraut, and fermented vegetables, like beets, carrots, daikon radishes, and other root vegetables. *Lacto* comes from lactic acid bacteria, not from milk products. However, fermented milk products are also desirable, including yogurt, kefir, and kumiss. They should be made from whole milk. Shun products that are made with milk powder, skim milk, reduced-fat milk, or milk substitutes.

Unless you are gluten-intolerant, consume whole-grain cereals and breads. If you are gluten-intolerant, there are whole grains that do not contain gluten, including quinoa, amaranth, teff, brown rice, wild rice, millet, undegerminated cornmeal, and buckwheat (not a true grain). It is difficult to find whole-grain crackers produced domestically, but a few brands are imported from Europe. Read labels carefully. Avoid packaged, ready-to-eat cereals.

Eat as wide a variety of foods as possible. By doing so, you will minimize the likelihood of developing a food allergy due to overconsumption of the same foods. Both corn and soybeans are major allergens, due to their overuse in the industrialized food supply. A variety of foods is more likely to offer a range of nutrients than a diet that is restricted to a limited number of foods. This problem is especially acute among extreme vegetarians, such as vegans, and those who consume only raw foods.

Remember that you are unique. Although everyone requires all essential nutrients, individual needs vary greatly. One diet does not suit everyone. The best discussion of uniqueness is in Dr. Roger J. Williams's *You Are Extraordinary* (1967). An appreciation of individual differences will guide you to a diet that suits you. Because of individual differences, there is a role for nutritional supplements. They help repair the damage from past faulty diets and supply nutrients low in the industrialized diet. Numerous studies show that many Americans are low in or have marginal intakes of many nutrients.

Eat slowly, in a relaxed setting, and enjoy your food. It has been shown that we obtain nutrients better from our food if we savor it. Eating when stressed is incompatible with good digestion. Whenever possible, eat in a social setting.

Drink adequate amounts of plain, unflavored water. Tap water is good in many communities. Don't buy into the fad of pricey bottled water unless the safety of your water supply is dubious.

Eat seasonally, insofar as possible. Grow some of your own food, if you can. Even a postage stamp–sized garden can grow an amazing amount of produce. Support community gardens and farmers' markets. Eat locally as much as you can. Foods shipped cross-country are no longer very fresh, and shipments require lots of energy, increasing our carbon footprint.

Is nutrition the whole answer to good health? Emphatically not. However, nutrition frequently is overlooked as an important factor, whereas drugs are suggested as the first option to "solve" a problem. Also, what is offered as preventive medicine is simplistic if you are told to "eat a balanced diet" and exercise. The concept may be sound, but it is never spelled out with any specificity. The balanced diet certainly is not the one officially endorsed by dietary guidelines and pyramids.

Along with a truly healthy diet, taking into consideration the suggestions I offered above, you need to incorporate other lifestyle factors: low stress, economic security, pleasant living quarters, accessibility to services, social connections, meaningful work beyond self, hobbies, mental stimulation, and taking time to relax and enjoy the experiences that each new day brings. Smell the flowers, or marvel at the spectacular sunset while you munch on a pear.

15

The Truth About Ageless Beauty

Kat James

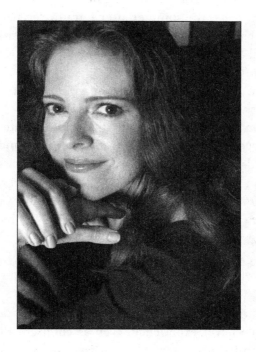

Kat James, author of the word-of-mouth best-seller *The Truth About Beauty: Transform Your Looks and Your Life from the Inside Out,* transformed herself beyond recognition after an eating disorder and resulting auto-immune disorders nearly took her life. Since 2000, her acclaimed Total Transformation® lifestyle programs have become nationally recognized for consistently producing extraordinary transformation success stories in people of all ages—not unlike her own. Website: www. informed beauty.com

We've all seen people who are inexplicably more vital in their gray years than many younger people are in their so-called prime. Genes play a part. So can the attractiveness of wisdom and self-knowledge. But from what I have experienced personally, and observed in my older program attendees, biochemistry is a very big player. Vitality is the universal aesthetic. It is where health and spirit meet. It can transcend the beauty of the features we were born with and make us more compelling at fifty than an "average person" (of average health) might be at twenty-nine.

About fifteen years ago, my then-eight-year-old niece pointed at a picture of me in 1984, the summer after I graduated from high school (deep into my battle with compulsive eating, and after many years of what I now call "denatured living") and said, "Aunt Kat, you looked like you were *fifty!*"

"No, Cecilia," I said, "that's just what we *think* fifty looks like. I'll never look that way again. Not even when I'm eighty."

I stumbled on my own fountain of youth quite unintentionally. Had I not been forced to address a life-threatening liver and autoimmune crisis in my mid-twenties, stemming from an eating disorder, I would never have been forced to open my mind to the world of information that would ultimately help me solve my own "Rubik's cube" of health issues, and show me my true physical potential. Without that wake-up call, I would likely have continued on a steady path of subclinical self-destruction and clung to that "denatured" lifestyle regimen that had created the fast-aging image in my mirror, and the deadly health consequences I was facing at twenty-four.

Today I live with a degree of peace in my body and peace with food that most people never experience, even as children. I'll never forget what life used to be like and might not have believed people if they'd told me such freedom was possible—unless they'd achieved it for themselves. My discoveries enabled me not only to preserve my own life in the face of a disease that is rarely cured, but to discern the array of biochemical issues behind my eating disorder and end my compulsive self-sabotage more than a decade ago. I have not had to work out, count calories, or even think about my body in order to "maintain" the size 10 dress size weight loss that ensued. It's amazing what happens when you stop torturing and start proactively supporting yourself on a cellular level.

DON'T FALL FOR COMMON DIETARY MYTHS

Every body is different. For example, studies suggest that people with healthy blood sugar metabolisms do better on high–complex carb, low-fat diets than those who are challenged with weight issues and metabolic syndrome. Because the latter now make up at least two-thirds of our country's population, I want to share my experience, having been a poster child for today's overweight and insulin-resistant norm—and gotten out alive and transformed.

I've adopted multiple eating styles over the course of my journey to health. When I moved to New York from Michigan in 1989, I literally learned what real food was (I grew up on nasty, processed food; iceberg lettuce salads; etc.). Then I evolved to whole-grain breads and pastas, and vegetarianism for several years. I thought I'd surely reached the pinnacle of healthy eating at that point, as I felt a huge difference in switching to whole grains (though it didn't affect my eating disorder one iota). But it was when I instinctively stopped eating flour and whole grains, and started eating a lot of good fats (nuts, avocados, and even organic butter), that my insulin-resistant body felt the most profound level of healing. Again, everyone's different, but by rejecting the popular dietary advice to avoid animal fats, dairy, eggs, and tropical oils, and to eat lots of whole grains, I've achieved the body, skin, and relationship with food I could only have dreamed of on my old dietary regimen.

DON'T BE TIMID WITH SUPPLEMENTS

I couldn't have turned my health around without supplements, and in fact, they likely saved my life. Not only did they repair my very sick liver, but they stoked my slow thyroid, totally transformed my skin, dramatically improved my moods, and healed the druglike reaction my body once had to food. Food alone did not do this for me. Forever downplayed because they're not patentable (read: profitable), supplements are, nonetheless, the safest and most powerful form of healing we have.

Expecting good information from your doctor about supplements is like asking your plumber about your electrical wiring. Don't ask what your doctor thinks about supplements. Ask what he *knows*. With a search engine, a couple of spare hours, and a little critical thinking, it's easy for a layperson to learn more than the average doctor knows about how supplements can benefit her own health.

BUCK THE BOOT-CAMP MENTALITY

I began to eat a "healthy" diet of natural foods and lots of grains in my early twenties. Yet, as a result of my exposure to the New York City high-fashion world as a makeup artist for magazines and celebrities, I had been deeply convinced that beauty and a beautiful body could only be achieved through hard work, self-deprivation, professional intervention, and keeping up with endless product trends. And then my own transformation (the only permanent one that left me at peace) challenged everything I'd long believed.

Few would question the value of this eternal tug-of-war we call "maintaining ourselves." But, believe it or not, we weren't meant to live that way. There is a force more powerful than our will that dictates how we treat ourselves—a force that, if ignored, will guarantee us a lifetime of struggle. But if this force were addressed, we could free ourselves of our struggles with both disease and self-sabotage, in this lifetime. It's called our biochemistry.

THE BEAUTY AND ANTI-AGING MYTHS

In all my years in the beauty field, which included working with older celebrities such as Martha Stewart, I'd become so adept at clever hair and wardrobe techniques to keep people from looking at my body or skin that I spent a fortune on cosmetics and wardrobe. At one point during the weight loss (health gain) process, I looked in mirror as I was applying my thick layer of foundation. Something made me stop and wash it off. In that moment I saw for the first time, around the age of thirty, what I was supposed to look like. Nature's intention. Something I had never even seen a hint of, even as a teen. I never covered my face with foundation again.

The myth I really want to bust is that you'll look better if you spend all your money on facials, moisturizers, hair removal, highlights, color cosmetics, and shoes, than if you spent a tenth of the cost on a collection of superstar supplements, and truly effective, nontoxic skin care products. Ultraconcentrated seaweed extract, vitamin C, and peptide-based serums are what I have found to be the most transforming topicals, along with internally taken fish oil; glucosamine (at least 1,500 mg a day) to inhibit and reverse age spots; "internal sunscreens" (that is, sunscreens that protect us from the inside out), such as lutein and cocoa flavonoids (which I like to eat in the form of very dark chocolate); targeted supplementation and bioidentical hormone-balancing measures to meet individual needs (and to address brain and mental health issues); as well as collagen drinks and hyaluronic acid supplements to plump the skin. With a strictly nonblood sugar–spiking, half-raw, and nutrient-dense diet included in that combo, you're guaranteed better skin than any department store regimen could ever deliver. And probably another ten or more vital years to your life.

EXPECT SOME UNEXPECTED NEW CHAPTERS TO BE ADDED TO YOUR LIFE

It's never too late to undergo a dramatic transformation. Over the years, I have seen so many people recover nearly lost chapters of prime life. One woman who attended my program in the spring of 2008 had this to say: "I never thought of myself as attractive. Today, at sixty-eight I am actually feeling beautiful for the first time. This ongoing recovery of health is like an inner secret. I am now actually excited for the future, instead of feeling washed up."

An executive in her late fifties had attended an earlier program and completely changed her habits, resulting in a lot of weight loss, shrinkage of her thyroid nodules, and blood lipid improvements. The only problem was that the better she took care of herself, the more her husband's self-health abuse became intolerable to her. Finally, he agreed to "get with the program" and actually came with her to another retreat. This, she says, has enabled her to envision longer, healthier retirement years together and has possibly saved her marriage, she says.

16

The Future of Anti-Aging Medicine

Ronald Klatz, MD, DO

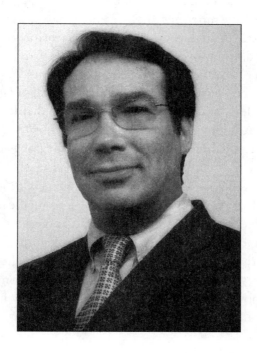

Ronald Klatz is the cofounder and president of the American Academy of Anti-Aging Medicine (A4M). He is the author of several books, including *121 Ways to Live 121 Years and More!* and *The Official Anti-Aging Revolution: Stop the Clock, Time is on Your Side for a Younger, Stronger, Happier You.* Address: 1510 West Montana Street; Chicago, IL 60614. Tel: 773-528-4333. Website: www.worldhealth.net

In the 1980s, I first coined the term *anti-aging medicine*. The origins of the anti-aging medical specialty can be traced directly to its two founding physicians, myself and Robert Goldman, MD, PhD, DO, FAASP (see his chapter, starting on p. 59). In August 1992, Dr. Goldman and I convened a meeting among a dozen physicians to discuss scientific breakthroughs making major inroads in identifying the mechanisms of deterioration and vulnerability to age-related diseases. In leading this group of medical pioneers, we introduced a new definition of aging. According to this new perspective, the frailties and physical and mental failures associated with normal aging are caused by physiological dysfunctions that, in many cases, can be altered by appropriate medical interventions. As an extension of this redefinition, I proposed an innovative model for health care that focused on the application of advanced scientific and medical technologies for the early detection, prevention, treatment, and reversal of age-related dysfunction, disorders, and diseases. Anti-aging medicine was born, and the American Academy of Anti-Aging Medicine (A4M) was established. I became the anti-aging movement's first physician and chief champion.

Anti-aging medicine, which is the fastest-growing medical specialty in the world, applies advanced scientific and medical technologies to the early detection, prevention, treatment, and reversal of age-related dysfunction, disorders, and diseases. It is a health care model promoting innovative science and research to extend the healthy life span in humans. As such, anti-aging medicine is based on principles of sound and responsible medical care, it is scientifically based, and it is well documented in leading medical journals.

THE ANTI-AGING MEDICAL CONCEPT

Today, cutting-edge therapies for life enhancement and potential life extension, available at top anti-aging clinics around the world, include the following:

- Exercise and lifestyle: Add 5–15 years
- Anti-aging drugs: Add 5–20 years
- High-tech biomedicine: Add 10–30 years

- Fasting and caloric restriction: Add 20–70 years

And the technologies of tomorrow add many new anti-aging approaches to the clinical arsenal:

- Advanced prospective diagnostics: Add 3–10 years
- Genetic screening and interventions: Add 3–10 years
- Stem cell therapeutics: Add 6–15 years
- Nanotechnology: Add 7–20 years
- Artificial organs: Add 8–20 years

So it is fully conceivable for the combined effect of existing and future biomedical technologies to extend the healthy human life span by upwards of sixty years.

Indeed, human life expectancy is not predetermined, finite, or immutable. In a study conducted by demographer J. R. Wilmoth and colleagues, the researchers found that in Sweden, the maximum age at death had risen from 100 years during the 1860s to about 108 years during the 1990s. They also observed that the increase in longevity has become expedited: Before 1969, the increase in maximum age at death increased 0.44 years per decade; since 1969, it has risen at the pace of 1.11 years per decade.

ANTI-AGING INTERVENTIONS OF TODAY

Today, extrapolating from hundreds of anti-aging research experiments conducted on nonhuman (animal) models, longevity could potentially be extended 20 to 300 percent via biomedical technologies already proven in the laboratory setting. Demographic studies show that, in humans, adoption of the anti-aging lifestyle contributes to optimal health by extending the healthy, productive life span by as much as thirty years.

As I outline them below, there are four key anti-aging interventions that every one of us can employ today to help reach the goal of the extended healthy human life span.

Lifestyle

Lifestyle is perhaps the most easily modifiable, proven anti-aging intervention. Recently, researchers from the Harvard School of Public Health found that the longest-living Americans are Asian-American women residing in Bergen County, New Jersey. They live longer than any other ethnic group in the United States, with an average life span of 91.1 years. By contrast, the Harvard team found that the shortest-living Americans are Native American populations in South Dakota, living an average of 66.5 years. The researchers identified several factors associated with the extraordinary longevity of the Asian-American women in Bergen County, namely: high median income; college education or better; occupations in management or professional settings; diet emphasizing fruits, vegetables, fish, and green tea; and lifestyle, including Eastern healing techniques.

Diet and Nutrition

Next, diet and nutrition have been found to play a profound role in longevity. Elderly Okinawans have among the lowest mortality rates in the world from a multitude of chronic diseases of aging and, as a result, enjoy not only what may be the world's longest life expectancy, but the world's longest health expectancy. Okinawans have an average life expectancy of eighty-two years, among the longest in the world. Their secrets: low caloric intake; a plant-based diet, high in vegetables and fruits; high intake of good fats (omega-3s, monounsaturated fats); high fiber intake; high flavonoid intake; and consumption of green tea.

Similarly, the Mediterranean diet has been found by numerous studies to contribute strongly to longevity. Featuring high consumption of grains, fruits, vegetables, legumes, and nuts; good fats (olive oil and omega-3 fatty acids); and a sparingly low intake of red meat, the Mediterranean diet correlates to a notably low incidence of chronic diseases and high life-expectancy rates. A 2003 study by researchers at Harvard Medical School found that people living in Mediterranean countries live longer. Resveratrol (found in red wine) and quercetin (in onions, apples, and olive oil) were turn-on genes that promote life extension.

Not only have scientists found that what we eat influences how long and how well we live, but they have also learned that how much we consume plays a major role as well. A team from Louisiana State University reported in 2006 on the findings from the first completed human study of the effect of calorie-restricted diets on life span, the Comprehensive Assessment of the Long Term Effects of Reducing Intake of Energy (CALERIE) study. It found that prolonged caloric restriction in humans reversed two of three biomarkers of longevity—fasting insulin level and core body temperature—and that it also reduced DNA damage and DNA fragmentation.

Stress Response

Third, we now know that the ability to cope with psychological stress factors into longevity. Researchers at the University of California–San Francisco found that chronic psychological stress is associated with accelerated shortening of telomeres on white blood cells. These shortened telomeres were found to correlate with a weakened immune system as well as an elevated risk of cardiovascular disease. The most-stressed study participants looked ten years older than their chronological age. Similarly, researchers from Tel Aviv University in Israel found that in otherwise healthy people, job stress was found to fuel the onset of type 2 diabetes. Employees who experienced job burnout were 1.8 times more likely to develop the condition. Stress was found to disrupt the body's ability to produce glucose.

Dietary Supplementation

Fourth, dietary supplementation has been found to be a strong contributor to both quality and quantity of life. Dr. Ranjit Chandra and colleagues from Memorial University in Newfoundland, administered a supplement containing eighteen vitamins, minerals, and trace elements to healthy men and women age sixty-five-plus, finding that:

1. Those who took the supplement showed "significant improvement in short-term memory, problem-solving ability, abstract thinking, and attention."

2. Nutritional supplementation "may be instrumental in preserving the anatomy and function of neurons and their appendages." As a result these men and women enhanced their capacities to live independently and without major disability.

3. The multivitamin, multimineral supplement improved immunity. The numbers of natural killer cells and helper T-cells, and the production of interleukin-2, all improved. Infection-related illness in those taking the supplement occurred at less than half the rate (23 days/year) compared to those who took placebo (48 days/year).

Source: R. K. Chandra, "Effect of vitamin and trace-element supplementation on cognitive function in elderly subjects." *Nutrition* 17, no. 9 (September 2001): 709–712.

ANTI-AGING INTERVENTIONS OF TOMORROW

We are now ushering in a new reality, in which seventy-five years old may well be considered middle age. We need only bridge the gap between the medical knowledge of today and the medical knowledge that we will have within our grasp by the year 2029. If medical knowledge doubles every 3.5 years or less, by 2029 we will know at least 256 times more than we know today. As a result, it is not impracticable nor improbable to expect that humankind will reach the point where we'll know how to substantially slow or perhaps even stop aging, and even eventually reset the clock of life itself. By the year 2029, we anticipate that science will enable us to achieve *practical immortality*—healthy human life spans of 150 years and beyond.

In my Model of Practical Immortality, we may consider the years from 2006 through 2029, collectively, as a Bridge to Practical Immortality, during which science will amass key knowledge in biomedical technologies that will enable 150-plus-year-long life spans.

I submit that the leading causes of death could be eliminated in the immediate future, were an all-out scientific effort mounted and the politics of disease-based medicine constrained. As such, I predict the following timetable for major medical breakthroughs during the period I call the Bridge to Practical Immortality:

• AIDS and Infectious Disease: Eliminated 2025

- Alzheimer's Disease: Eliminated 2015
- Cancer: Eliminated 2021
- Diabetes: Eliminated 2017
- Heart Disease: Eliminated 2016

To paraphrase the Swedish political leader and former secretary-general of the United Nations, Dag Hjalmar Agne Carl Hammarskjold (1905–1961), "Never look [back] to test the ground before taking your next step; only he who keeps his eye fixed on the far horizon will find the right road."

17

Diet and Adaptogens

Marcus Laux, ND

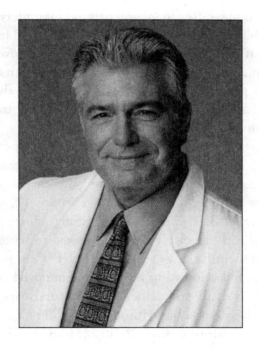

Marcus Laux is a licensed naturopathic physician, a clinical professor, and a recognized leader in the field of alternative health care. He writes *Dr. Marcus Laux's Naturally Well Today* newsletter. Address: Healthy Living Communications, LLC, P.O. Box 1934, San Ramon, CA 94583. Website: www.drmarcuslaux.com

Your health is the greatest of gifts in life. It's not money, fame, or toys, but the true treasure is the freedom and comfort of optimal health. It is a most fortuitous inheritance, indeed, and one, like other precious wealth, that you can either protect and enhance, or squander too easily into bankruptcy. To have the ability to climb or slide, walk or skip, swim or dance—being fully functional, flexible, and free—is living with healthy vitality. Most of us take our natural health gift for granted, until we are reminded of its ease, grace, and the amazing joy it confers; until, that is, we are limited by an ache, a cold, or a cough.

This is the simple, self-evident and paramount understanding we all should fully embrace much sooner rather than later. Health may be a given today, but it is not a lifelong guarantee. However, you have a major role to play in your health's future. Studies with twins show us that perhaps 75 percent of the odds of living well into the nineties and beyond are determined by modifiable factors we control and, therefore, can change.

Two recent studies add more proof that you are never too old to change, and it's never too late to start, but the sooner the better, the sooner the easier, safer, and more lasting gains can be yours.

Both studies were reported in the February 11, 2008 issue of *Archives of Internal Medicine.* The first study showed that healthy lifestyles in our early elderly years were linked to better odds of living to ninety in men. Exactly as it should be! The second study found that while some folks do live to be over one hundred years old without major disease, many still achieve this century mark and continue to stay active with disease but without its disability. Lifestyle support can curb disease and prevent disability. Lifestyle effects can kill or cure, and even the small transgressions you ignore can act like water slowly eroding away your rock of solid health. You are in charge, so take the reins and responsibility: Your doctor is only a supporting actor.

While health is in part DNA-directed by our genes, it's also true, and more to my point, that what we do—moment to moment, day after day, consciously and unconsciously—also greatly determines our genetic wellness profile. So much of our genetics is not fixed and immutable, but rather wonderfully flexible and adaptable, and highly trainable. Our genes can respond rapidly and decisively to help secure our good health or hinder our healing, depending on how we experience the influences and pressures applied in our life. From our habits, diet, and lifestyle, our daily dose of healthy living helps direct our genes' expression of safety and health; alternatively, an unhealthy lifestyle can promote a dangerous slide toward dysfunction, degeneration, and disease.

We can turn on our genes for excellent health and turn off our genes for disease now! Smart choices and living within nature's laws can transform our health destiny. In fact, nothing else we can do or take can make our quality of life and future outlook appear as bright! Habits can heal, and daily habits change and charge our genes for life!

Enjoyable health and rewarding longevity are created, renewed, and fully delivered through your daily life. Your habits and lifestyle choices do more for your health than any one factor—period. It's about getting back to basics. It's about caring for yourself, as prevention pays off bigger and better than any "after the fact" treatment ever can. No wonder drug or magical potion can do for you what you can do for yourself.

DIET'S ROLE IN LONGEVITY

You have to eat to live, so really eat to live. Eat organic as much as feasible. You are what you eat, so make sure it is excellent! Don't be fooled by genetically modified foods. No matter what is publicized, the behind-the-scenes safety and health data looks bad to terrible. Avoid genetically modified foods, cloned and chemicalized foods. Healthy and nutritious produce is grown naturally, not fabricated. There is no other way. Yes, it's common sense, but it appears as if common sense is less common these days.

This next item should have been in your folks' owner's manual, but I realize that many got lost early on. At every meal, eat a combination of protein, fat, and carbohydrates for lasting energy that burns your food as "fuel" and does not pack on the pounds as fat. This single meal menu makeover magic can save your life and waistline forever. It's not just calories, but they need to be within reason. It's not just one food group to eat or avoid, but combining them together helps your metabolism hum along strong, so you eat well, keep your energy up, and your weight down. It's not magic, but it is basic metabolism.

In traditional cultures worldwide, every meal, including breakfast, lunch, and dinner, is prepared with an assortment of the three major macronutrient players. In the United States, that's not the case, and it is one of the reasons for our growing rates of diabetes, heart disease, and obesity.

When you wake up in the morning after sleeping eight hours, you awake with a fat-burning, calorie-crunching metabolism. This is our normal fat-burning metabolic mode. You want to stay in this metabolic mode all day to ensure plenty of energy and lean body mass. If you wake up and have nothing more than prepackaged cereal and orange juice for breakfast, you effectively shut off this metabolic machinery and kick-start the less effective calorie-storage mode. But, if you had an egg, smoked salmon, butter, rice or oatmeal, tea and tomato juice, then you could have even enjoyed more calories, and still burned that energy off—without turning on the fat-storage mechanism. You can keep your metabolism burning calories throughout the day and night. It is how we are designed to operate; it's just not how we have been nutritionally educated. We are very far away from our roots—both our genetic legacy as well as the soil's soul. Returning to our ancestral diet and nature's more nutritious organic foods will do more than all the drugs and doctors ever could.

Each meal and every snack is best prepared with a contribution of proteins, fats, and carbohydrates. This one big change can have a tremendous effect on energy levels, while naturally trimming your waistline. We know that appetite suppression is best accomplished with more protein consumed at the meal. Ghrelin is the only known appetite-stimulating hormone, and it is secreted by the stomach. Eating fat allows its levels to remain fairly high, and while carbohydrates can lower it temporarily, it rebounds back higher than its starting baseline. Both scenarios are bad news! A carbohydrate-induced ghrelin rebound can make you eat more food, more often, and if you choose to eat carbohydrates again, well, you start to store those calories as fat, instead of burning them for energy, in a vicious cycle of crash and burn. This can spiral quickly into glucose dysregulation, weight gain, metabolic syndrome, and prediabetes in a matter of weeks.

Ensuring more of a protein presence at each meal (and snacks), combined with some quality fats and complex carbohydrates, will help you suppress ghrelin levels more effectively and longer. This is not only smart for suppressing this appetite accelerator, but it will help your metabolism function better. This combination of macronutrients on your plate ensures a controlled and lower insulin level.

As you span the globe, it's eye-openingly obvious that other cultures eat very differently than we do. And, that most of them are healthier, thinner, and more robustly energetic at every age. Whether in Belize or Belgium, Guam or Greece, the composition of each and every meal helps guide healthy metabolism and functional longevity. This is the dietary macronutrient menu found in most traditional cultures.

ADAPTOGENS AND LONGEVITY

After any menu mending, next consider an alliance with an adaptogen. If you consider only one nutritional supplement to adopt, I highly recommend an adaptogen. No other class of nutritional or herbal support can offer more health prevention and metabolic protection for living well and thriving in spite of today's challenging world.

The word *adaptogen* was coined by a Soviet scientist who was on assignment to find ways to enhance performance and productivity without dangerous stimulants. While the adaptogenic label to describe their effects is relatively new, the concept is commonly found in traditional herbal medicines worldwide, including the Chinese, ayurvedic, and the Native American. They are powerful tonic herbs with the ability to restore and rebalance health.

No other botanical bounty has as many health-promoting, stress-busting, and body-balancing benefits to offer. They are believed to function synergistically through the hypothalamic/pituitary/adrenal axis and the sympathoadrenal system. Adaptogens support the integrated regulation of our body systems, especially the endocrine, immune, and nervous systems. This helps modulate our stress response, keeping us cool under fire, and more balanced in an increasingly unbalanced world, regardless of whether our stress stems from an environmental, emotional, or physical source.

Adaptogens are very special plants with exceptional qualities. These plants mostly grow in the most extreme and inhospitable environments around the world, including the coldest, the highest, and most desolate UV-scorched places on earth. Their ability to survive and thrive where little else can is the quality they seem to transfer and ignite in us when they are properly consumed.

Examples abound, with better-known representatives including Panax ginseng, Eleutrococcus senticoccus, Shisandra chinensis, Ashwagandha (Withania somnifera), Suma (Pfaffia paniculata), Maca, Reshi (Ganoderma lucidum) Coryceps, Codonopsis pilosula, Holy basil (Ocimum sanctum) Rhodiola rosea, Jiaogulan (Gynostemma pentaphylla), and Licorice (Glycyrrhiza glabra).

The best Panax ginseng available is made from six-year-old Korean roots that have the most ginsenoside content known among the world's ginsengs. Accept no substitutes here, as way too many products tested fall short of the mark of this restorative herbal treasure's active constituents, if they contain any at all! Once you have experienced an authentic root extract, you'll know firsthand its life-enhancing power for the mind and body.

While Panax may be too stimulating for some, Eleutrococcus or Maca are nonstimulatory adaptogens, whereas Ashwagandha can be quite relaxing in its effects. You will want to explore and find your best personal match.

We can use all the help we can get, and nature has provided us with just what we need. Mend your menu as needed, and adopt adaptogens to live the promise and potential that lives in us all.

18

The Dangers of Grains

Shari Lieberman, PhD, CNS, FACN

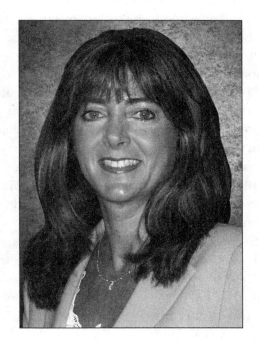

Shari Lieberman is a nutrition scientist and the best-selling author of *The Real Vitamin and Mineral Book* as well as *Dare to Lose* and other nutrition books for "real" people. Her latest book, coauthored with Linda Segall, is *The Gluten Connection* (2007). Tel: 212-439-8728. Website: www.drshari.net

I am a nutrition scientist. I help people eat right to be healthy.

As a private practitioner, I am frequently the professional of last resort. People come to me, often through medical referral, after they have unsuccessfully tried other, often easier, remedies for their health problems.

It was through these cases of last resort that I became intrigued with a condition that my research has shown plagues about 30 percent—or more—of the American population. It is a condition that has the ability to hide behind a variety of symptoms, which makes it difficult to diagnose correctly. And without the correct diagnosis, medical doctors tend to prescribe harsh pharmaceuticals that often cause even more complicating problems than the original disease.

The condition? *Gluten sensitivity*, also known as *gluten intolerance.*

Gluten is a protein found in wheat, barley, and rye. People who are sensitive to gluten have an autoimmune reaction to it: They are unable to digest the protein as "normal" people do. Their body recognizes gluten as an enemy and tries to fight it off.

You may actually have a low level of gluten sensitivity without identifiable and easily recognizable symptoms or with symptoms so mild that you do not pay attention to them. Feeling less than 100 percent may have become "normal."

Unfortunately, autoimmune reactions are often cumulative: They get worse with additional introductions of the offending food. Ultimately, in the case of gluten, the autoimmune reaction can lead to celiac disease (CD).

Researchers and doctors have associated gluten with celiac disease for more than fifty years. But it was the *only* problem they identified with gluten. They did not grasp (and many still do not, unfortunately) that the culprit behind celiac disease could be causing a myriad of other problems long before it manifested itself as a disease of the gut.

Until recently, MDs and medical researchers thought CD was rare. In 2003, however, researchers at the University of Maryland conducted an extensive survey of more than 13,000 people and found that 1 out of 133 people in the general population has CD.

But many more than 1 out of 133 people are gluten-sensitive. Think of it this way: CD is the "extreme edition" of gluten sensitivity. People can be gluten-sensitive but *not* have CD, but *all* patients who have CD are gluten-sensitive.

As a nutritionist, I recognize that people eat foods that nature never meant for them to eat. In today's society this is especially true. Most food we have available to consume is processed—changed from the way that nature made it. Biochemists have changed the seeds from which plants are grown. And food manufacturers have introduced additives to the foods they sell to improve texture and extend shelf life.

The majority of people can tolerate (and even enjoy) processed foods. But some people cannot.

And it is often this minority of people who come to nutritionists for help. As we work with them, we examine their diets for suspect foods, including the common allergens of milk, eggs, fish, shellfish, tree nuts, peanuts, wheat, soybeans, and nightshades. Then we work with them to modify their diets and eliminate troublesome foods and their derivatives and introduce wholesome nutrition, including appropriate supplementation, to make up for possible deficiencies caused by their physical conditions.

It was through this course of action that I discovered the powerful effect gluten can have—and the even more dramatic effect that taking gluten *out* of a diet can have on a person's health. Today, when I work with patients, gluten sensitivity is high on my list of possible causes of their problems because it affects so many people in so many ways.

A CHAMELEONLIKE DISEASE

Gluten-sensitivity is a chameleonlike disease that can develop in many different, unsuspected ways. It can masquerade as any of the following conditions:

- **Skin diseases**, such as dermatitis herpetiformis, psoriasis, eczema, acne, and hives.

- **Neurological disorders**, including ataxia, severe headaches, and behavioral problems, such as attention deficit disorder and autism.

- **Other autoimmune diseases**, such as lupus, multiple sclerosis, diabetes, scleroderma, thyroid disease, rheumatoid arthritis, and ankylosing spondylitis.

- **Digestive disorders**, including irritable bowel syndrome (IBS), irritable bowel disease (IBD), Crohn's disease, ulcerative colitis, proctitis, gastroesophageal reflux, ulcers, giardiasis, and celiac disease.

- **Undiagnosed diseases and conditions**, like catch-all conditions such as chronic fatigue syndrome, fibromyalgia, unexplained weight loss or gain, anemia, chronic infection, and asthma.

A FEW OF MY MIRACLE CASES

I personally have treated individuals who have suffered with many of these different conditions. When I put them on a gluten-free diet, their symptoms disappeared. I could fill pages with case studies that illustrate the miracles of going gluten-free; however, consider these few:

- In the early 1980s, a fourteen-year-old Canadian girl suffering from Crohn's disease (a chronic inflammation of the digestive tract) was brought to me for help. Pharmaceutical intervention was limited back then, and the drugs that were available had been ineffective for this girl. The doctors advised removing part of her colon, which would remove necrotic tissue but not halt the disease. Her parents wanted to avoid this last-ditch effort. I put the girl on a gluten-free diet. Within thirty days, *all* her symptoms resolved.

- A young woman in her early twenties was suffering from type 1 diabetes, previously known as juvenile diabetes. Despite taking insulin and watching her diet carefully, she could not control her blood sugar levels; as a result, she experienced diabetes-related problems, including retinopathy. I put her on a high-fiber diet that included beans, lentils, and oatmeal. Her condition stabilized, except when she ate oatmeal (*without* added sugar). Then her blood sugar would skyrocket to more than 200. I put her on a gluten-free diet that included an absence of oats. Oats in themselves do not contain gluten, but they are often contaminated with gluten, because they are generally processed in the same plants that process wheat and are often grown in the same fields where wheat has been grown. Within two weeks, the patient found she could go days without taking insulin to regulate her blood sugar. And after several months, even her retinopathy substantially improved.

- A distraught mother brought me her ten-year-old daughter, who exhibited behavioral problems characteristic of a child with attention deficient disorder (ADD). She could not concentrate or sit still, and she was impulsive. Her schoolwork was greatly affected by her inability to concentrate. The mother had tried everything except Ritalin, a medication that works as a stimulant on the central nervous system and is often prescribed to calm ADD children. The mother did not want to expose her child to the risks involved with pharmaceuticals. Among her attempts at solving the girl's behavior problems was the Feingold diet, which eliminates foods with artificial coloring and flavoring, synthetic sweeteners, and the artificial preservatives BHA, BHT, and TBHQ. The diet is effective with many ADD children, but not with this girl.

  Although this child did not have any physical symptoms to suggest a sensitivity to gluten (such as digestive problems), I put her on a gluten-free diet. Six weeks later, the mother called to tell me her daughter had "aced" a math test and her behavior and learning were so greatly improved that she was being moved from a special education class to a regular class! The change in the girl was dramatic.

- I was the "last stop" for a four-year-old boy who was developmentally delayed and was diagnosed with a failure to thrive. He could not talk, but he could scream, which he did incessantly. Screaming was how he communicated with the world. I put the boy on a gluten-free diet, accompanied by a dairy-free diet. Within two weeks, the parents cried tears of happiness as they told me that not only had his behavior improved, but he had also spoken his first words! And he was already gaining weight. That case happened twenty-five years ago. The "boy" remains gluten-free to this day and is a normal young man.

- A thirty-year-old patient suffering from early-stage lupus asked for help. One of her primary symptoms was a "wolf mask" (discoloration on the face). After one month of being on a gluten-free diet, her skin cleared up, and her lupus went into full clinical remission.

- A woman with later-stage multiple sclerosis (MS) came to me for guidance. Although she had neurological damage and her left leg was impaired, she continued to exercise daily, determined to fight the disease that kept progressing. When she went on a gluten-free diet, the neurological progression stopped. Her damaged left leg regained some of its feeling, and her right leg returned to normal function. Even more important, her vision was restored! The diet stopped the MS's progression.

- Perhaps one of the most visibly dramatic improvements I've ever seen was the case of a young man who had been diagnosed with Darier's disease, a rare psoriasislike genetic skin condition that covers the person with a scaly rash. This young man had the rash from head to toe. The condition was so extreme that he would not wear T-shirts or shorts. He kept as much skin covered as possible to avoid embarrassing stares. I put him on a gluten-free and dairy-free diet. In less than six months, his skin cleared up completely. He even started going to the beach!

These case studies are convincing, but even more convincing is research showing that gluten is the culprit in these types of conditions and many more.

THE SOLUTION

You may not suffer from MS, lupus, diabetes, or eczema, but if you suspect that you (or someone close to you) may be gluten-sensitive because of chronic heartburn or mysterious bouts of diarrhea or other gastrointestinal problems, you can take action.

1. **Research gluten sensitivity.** Read about what it is, how it may be manifested, what the solution is (a gluten-free diet), and how the quality of your life would improve by avoiding gluten, should you actually be gluten-sensitive.

2. **Go a gluten-free diet.** This means you eliminate *everything* with gluten in it. (No cheating!) Go through your pantry, freezer, and refrigerator and check labels for gluten by looking for the words *wheat, barley,* or *rye.* (Note: Malt, used for flavoring in cereals, among other foods, is made from barley. Hence, products with malt contain gluten as well.)

3. **Go easy on the veggies.** If you have gastrointestinal problems, you may not be able to tolerate salads or raw or al dente vegetables initially, because of gastrointestinal inflammation. Introduce these vegetables slowly and judiciously once your symptoms have been alleviated.

4. **Drink water.** Stay away from carbonated drinks. They may cause gas.

5. **Take supplements.** Dietary supplementation gives recovery a boost. Use supplements in three stages:

Stage 1: Take multinutrients as well as the major antioxidants the body requires, including multivitamins, fish oil (approximately 2–3 grams a day), and coenzyme Q_{10} (100–200 mg per day). Take these stage 1 supplements for two or three weeks, until your symptoms have subsided.

State 2: Continue stage 1 supplementation. After two or three weeks, add vitamin C (1,000–4,000 mg, buffered and nonacidic) and quercetin (500–2,000 mg).

Stage 3: About one month into the gluten-free diet, you may begin the third stage of supplementation, which aids in the restoration of the intestine. Add acidophilus and other beneficial microorganisms (L. casei GG, 1 or 2 capsules daily [different supplements have different potencies, so follow label directions]; S. boulardii, 500 mg each day), glutamine (500–3,000 mg of L-glutamine), phosphatidylcholine (for collagen deposition and stricture formation, 100–300 mg daily), fiber (1 or 2 tablespoons of fiber supplement), and other anti-inflammatories (as needed).

Wheat is considered the staff of life, but if you are gluten-sensitive, it is a real danger to your health. But giving up wheat—the main source of gluten—is not the end of the world: You can still enjoy eating foods you enjoy because there are gluten-free versions of almost everything you like.

Beware the grain danger, and take cautionary steps to protect yourself. You'll be healthier for your new habits.

19

Homocysteine, B Vitamins, and Prevention of Disease

Kilmer S. McCully, MD

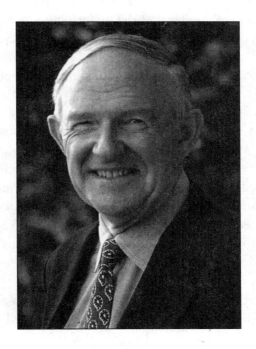

Kilmer McCully is one of the leading nutritionally oriented research physicians in the world. Dr. McCully developed the homocysteine theory of cardiovascular disease, and he is the author of *Reverse Heart Disease Now, The Heart Revolution,* and other books. Address: Pathology and Laboratory Medicine Service, VA Medical Center, 1400 Veterans of Foreign Wars Parkway, West Roxbury MA 02132. E-mail: Kilmer.mccully @med.va.gov orty years ago, I began a study of children with vascular disease—stroke, hardening of the arteries, and heart disease—and newly discovered diseases of metabolism involving the amino acid homocysteine. This study showed that accumulation of homocysteine in the blood of the children with these diseases causes vascular disease by damaging the lining of blood vessels and increasing the formation of blood clots within arteries and veins. Because homocysteine metabolism is controlled by the B vitamins—folic acid, vitamin B_{12}, and vitamin B_6, both in these children with inherited diseases and in normal subjects without disease—I suggested in my scientific articles and books for the general reader that the underlying cause of vascular disease in developed countries is related to dietary deficiencies of these vitamins.

My discoveries concerning the biochemical origin of vascular disease and diseases of aging were the culmination of my lifelong interest in biochemistry, genetics, molecular biology, medicine, and pathology. As a student majoring in chemistry at Harvard College, I was fortunate to study the biochemistry of cholesterol with two prominent professors, Louis Fieser and Konrad Bloch. As a student at Harvard Medical School, I studied steroid hormone metabolism, and my postdoctoral fellowship training concentrated on the biochemistry, molecular biology and genetics of amino acids and proteins. This fellowship experience was guided by the outstanding scientists Giulio Cantoni, Paul Zamecnik, Guido Pontecorvo, and James Watson.

After completing my residency in pathology at Massachusetts General Hospital, this prior fellowship experience enabled me in 1968 to understand the significance and origin of the advanced vascular disease that I discovered in children with homocystinuria. Because my discovery of the relation of homocysteine to vascular disease was not acceptable to investigators promoting the conventional cholesterol/fat hypothesis, I was forced to leave Harvard Medical School after eleven years of teaching, practice, and research. Fortunately, I was able to continue my investigation of homocysteine and disease in 1981 at the VA Medical Center in Providence, and since 2001 at the VA Medical Center in Boston.

HOMOCYSTEINE THEORY OF ARTERIOSCLEROSIS

In 1968 I discovered that two children with homocystinuria, caused by different inherited diseases of homocysteine metabolism, had died with advanced arteriosclerosis, hardening of the arteries. One child was an eight-year-old boy with mental retardation, dislocated ocular lenses, and mild abnormalities of his leg and breastbone, who suffered from sudden paralysis and coma and died at Massachusetts General Hospital in 1933. The autopsy revealed arteriosclerosis of the carotid artery with thrombosis and a massive stroke of one half of his brain, as discussed in a case presentation published in the *New England Journal of Medicine*. In 1965, pediatricians discovered the disease homocystinuria in a niece of this boy, and her mother recalled that the girl's uncle died with a similar disease in 1933, as described in the case report. The disease in these children is caused by an abnormal enzyme requiring vitamin B_6 that leads to a buildup of homocysteine within the plasma.

When I restudied this archival case from 1933, I became fascinated with the possibility that elevated levels of homocysteine actually caused the fatal arteriosclerosis and stroke in this child. Several months later I was able to restudy a second case of homocystinuria. This second child was a two-month-old baby boy who had died of pneumonia and failure to thrive. When I studied the arteries of this baby, I was astonished to discover advanced arteriosclerosis with extensive damage and plaque scattered throughout the body. I immediately realized that the amino acid homocysteine was responsible for the damage to the artery lining and blood clots occurring in these two children by a direct effect on the cells and tissues of the arteries. In this second case a different enzyme, dependent on folic acid and vitamin B_{12}, was abnormal, causing elevation of homocysteine in the plasma. Because of the different pattern of metabolism in the two cases, I reasoned that homocysteine elevation was the common feature accounting for the advanced vascular disease with thrombosis, stroke, and generalized arteriosclerosis.

In my experiments with rabbits I was able to confirm that high doses of homocysteine, given by injection or by feeding, produced arteriosclerosis in the arteries and, in a few animals, fatal thrombosis of the veins with embolism of blood clots to the lungs. In one experiment I was able to prevent the blood clots and fatal embolism by giving vitamin B_6 to the rabbits. In my experiments with cultured skin cells from a child with homocystinuria, I discovered a new pathway of metabolism of homocysteine to sulfate, the end product of metabolism of the amino acid methionine, which is the only metabolic precursor of homocysteine. My experiments with cultured cancer cells led to the discovery of a characteristic abnormality of homocysteine metabolism, the failure to convert the anhydride of homocysteine (homocysteine thiolactone) to sulfate. In subsequent years I discovered a compound called thioretinaco, containing homocysteine thiolactone, vitamin A, and vitamin B_{12}, which prevents cancer formation and cancer growth in mice and prevents arteriosclerosis in rats.

Because of these new observations in children with homocystinuria, production of arteriosclerosis by homocysteine in animals, and abnormalities of homocysteine metabolism in cell culture experiments, I proposed in 1975 a new theory of the origin of vascular disease called the homocysteine theory of arteriosclerosis. Very simply, this theory states that excess homocysteine produces arteriosclerosis by a toxic effect of the amino acid on cellular metabolism. Therefore, any means to lower plasma homocysteine, such as increased B vitamins, folic acid, vitamin B_{12}, and vitamin B_6 in the diet, will prevent vascular disease caused by homocysteine.

THE HEART REVOLUTION DIET

In order to explain the homocysteine theory of arteriosclerosis and to make the theory useful to the general reader, I published two books, *The Homocysteine Revolution* in 1997, and *The Heart Revolution* in 1999. In these books I explain how to use the principles of the theory to prevent disease. Keeping blood levels of homocysteine as low as possible through optimal nutrition will prevent damage to arteries and the complications of arteriosclerosis—heart disease, stroke, amputations, and kidney failure.

Optimal nutrition is lifelong consumption of a diet that provides abundant B vitamins—folic acid, vitamin B_{12}, and vitamin B_6—to keep homocysteine levels in the optimal range, 6–8 micromoles per liter.

Highly processed foods are deficient in vitamins B_6 and folic acid because the traditional methods of food processing—milling of grains to flour, commercial canning, use of chemical additives—destroy these sensitive vitamins. Vitamin B_{12} is present only in foods of animal origin—meats, seafood, dairy foods—and an optimal diet contains an abundance of these foods. The Heart Revolution diet consists of fresh meats, seafood, whole grains, and fresh vegetables and fruits, with a minimum of processed foods. Thus this optimal diet is virtually identical to traditional diets of indigenous or aboriginal peoples, as discovered by Weston Price, the twentieth-century dentist who observed the preventive effect of traditional diets on heart disease, tooth decay, infectious disease, and mental illness. This optimal diet also resembles the so-called Paleolithic diet that humankind evolved with over millions of years. The exceptions are grains and dairy foods that were introduced with the Agricultural Revolution twelve thousand years ago.

The great advantage of the Heart Revolution diet is that it provides many of the nutrients that, in addition to B vitamins, help to prevent vascular disease. Some of these nutrients are fish oil, containing omega-3 unsaturated oils; vitamins D and A; ubiquinone (CoQ_{10}); benzoquinone (vitamin K_2); beneficial phytochemicals; and the minerals magnesium, potassium, calcium, selenium, and other trace minerals.

The other great advantage of the Heart Revolution diet is that, because it largely eliminates processed foods, it provides little or none of the deleterious nutrients and artificial additives that contribute to chronic diseases of aging. Some of these deleterious dietary factors are foods containing soy products, fluoridated water, drugs containing fluorine, trans fats from hydrogenated oils, monosodium glutamate (MSG), aspartame and sucralose, oxidized forms of cholesterol, and the oxycholesterols.

Soy foods contain toxic proteins and phytoestrogenic substances that cause hypothyroidism, infertility, poor digestion, allergic reactions, and poor absorption of minerals. Fluoridated water from natural or added fluorides causes accelerated aging, hip fractures, increased risk of cancer, and dental and skeletal fluorosis. Drugs containing fluorine, such as statins, antidepressants, and certain corticosteroids, for example, are associated with multiple toxic side effects and should be avoided.

Trans fats from hydrogenated oils are associated with increased risk of stroke and heart disease, and excessive plant oils containing omega-6 oils are associated with increased risk of inflammatory disease and cancer. A recent analysis of scientific studies for the World Health Organization has implicated MSG and related forms of glutamic acid in susceptibility to obesity, diabetes, brain damage, cataracts, and abnormal brain development. The amount of MSG entering the food supply through hydrolyzed protein extracts, beef or malt flavoring, or direct addition of glutamate compounds is unknown because there is no labeling requirement by industry or governmental agencies.

Other potentially toxic but ubiquitous additives are aspartame, which releases methanol when heated, and sucralose, which contains synthetic chlorine derivatives of sugars. Oxidized forms of cholesterol, known as oxycholesterols, are formed within animal foods during processing, heating, or cooking. Some examples are spray-dried egg yolks, powdered milk, and fried foods, such as chicken, fish, and potatoes cooked in hot vegetable oils. The oxycholesterols in these foods cause plaque formation in the arteries of monkeys and other experimental animals within twenty-four hours of feeding or injection. By contrast, highly purified cholesterol protected from oxygen is an exceptionally effective antioxidant that protects arteries of these animals from damage and plaque formation.

PREVENTION OF DISEASE

Lifelong consumption of the Heart Revolution diet provides the correct quantity and balance of nutrients (proteins, fats, carbohydrates) and micronutrients (vitamins, minerals, phytochemicals) that are needed for healthy gestation, birth, development, healthful maturity, and aging. By avoiding processed foods, such as white flour; protein extracts; excessive sugars and oils; and canned, bleached, or preserved foods, the amount of healthful fresh foods will be dramatically increased. Typical Americans eat as much as 75 percent of their calories from nutritionally empty processed foods. By eating six to ten servings per day of fresh vegetables and fruits, two to three servings of whole grains or legumes, and two to three servings of fresh fish, poultry, meat, eggs, or other dairy foods per day, the amount of dietary

B vitamins will be adequate, homocysteine levels will be kept in the safe range (less than 8), and chronic diseases of aging will be prevented. The results are radiant physical and mental health and a long, productive life.

Some convincing evidence of the effectiveness of a diet providing abundant B vitamins was obtained from the Nurses' Health Study. In this study 80,000 nurses were followed for ten years. Those nurses who consumed in their diet more than 350 micrograms of folic acid and 3.5 milligrams of vitamin B_6 per day had significantly reduced risk of death and disability from coronary heart disease. In the Framingham Heart Study, the elderly participants who had the highest blood levels of the B vitamins had the lowest homocysteine levels and the lowest risk of vascular disease and stroke. Many other studies over the years support these dramatic findings.

As shown by the Centers for Disease Control (CDC), the death rate from heart disease reached a peak in the 1950s, and since then there has been a marked decline in mortality from this cause. The traditional risk factors—smoking, lack of exercise, blood cholesterol, fat in the diet—are unable to explain this decline. In fact, during the past two decades there has been an ominous increase in obesity and diabetes, even in children, that is related to the high-carbohydrate, low-fat diet promulgated by the "authorities." A likely explanation of the decline in heart disease mortality in the twentieth century is the addition of synthetic folic acid and vitamin B_6, beginning in the 1960s, in the form of supplements to cereals.

In 1998, the FDA mandated fortification of flour and refined grains with folic acid to combat birth defects (neural-tube defects) in children of mothers with dietary deficiency of folic acid. Follow-up studies confirmed significant reductions in these birth defects in the United States and Canada. Recent studies by the CDC showed that, beginning in 1998, the decline in stroke mortality in the United States and Canada declined at a tenfold more rapid rate, compared with England and Wales, where there was no fortification with folic acid and no change in stroke mortality. The Framingham Heart Study showed that folic acid fortification in 1998 led to a doubling of blood folate levels and a 15 percent decline in blood homocysteine levels in participants, compared with studies in the same subjects before 1996.

Are supplements of B vitamins helpful in prevention of disease? Recent studies showed that subjects with advanced vascular disease (stroke, heart disease, diabetes, kidney failure) did not benefit from moderate to high doses of B vitamins over periods of one to three years, even though homocysteine levels were lowered. However, recent studies of stroke mortality showed that there was a significant decrease in stroke, particularly among those with no prior disease, as well as a lowering of homocysteine levels more than 25 percent. A recent comprehensive analysis of genetic influences, observational studies, and intervention studies concluded that lowering homocysteine levels by an optimal diet, such as the Heart Revolution diet, and an optimal intake of B vitamins is associated with a 12 percent reduction in risk of heart disease and a 25 percent reduction in risk of stroke.

20

The Amazing Benefits of Goji Berries

Earl Mindell, RPh, PhD

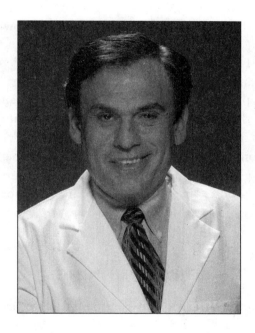

Earl Mindell is an internationally recognized expert on nutrition, drugs, vitamins, and herbal remedies. He is the author of *The Vitamin Bible for the 21st Century, Prescription Alternatives,* and many other books. Website: drmindell.com 'm a big fan of a berry that comes from a plant known to science as *Lycium barbarum L*—the goji berry. I sometimes call it the "Himalayan health secret," as it has been an integral part of the medical system of the very healthy, long-lived Himalayan people for centuries. Discovering and investigating this superfood has been a huge source of inspiration for me. I feel almost as though this is the discovery to which my whole career as a health educator and researcher has been leading all these years.

Goji isn't exactly a secret anymore; the number of Westerners who are using goji to help restore or promote good health is on the rise. It was bound to happen, because the science on this berry has hit critical mass. Still, I'd wager that most people don't know about goji, or if they do, that they don't grasp the full breadth and depth of the health potential of this food.

I'd like to start with a quick review/overview of goji history, biochemistry, and the general direction of the research, and then fill you in on some of the latest developments in the scientific investigation of this remarkable red fruit. Personally, I wouldn't even consider removing it from its rightful place in my daily regimen, right alongside my multivitamin/mineral supplement, workouts, and diet of nutrient-dense foods. Once you've shared in that knowledge, I hope you'll feel the same way about goji—a true superfood if ever there was one.

GOJI'S BEGINNINGS

About 70 million years ago, two continental plates slowly but inexorably drifted toward each other, until their edges met. They pushed and pushed against each other until, finally, the force caused a cataclysm that thrust skyward the highest peaks on earth: the Himalayas. Even today, those plates continue to crush toward one another, causing the mountains to become a few millimeters taller each year.

These mountains form a tremendous ridge that cuts through Asia, dividing the Indian subcontinent from the Tibetan plateau. The range's name is from a Sanskrit word that means the "abode of snow." This mountain range has over one hundred peaks that are higher than

7,200 meters—that's about 23,600 feet! The Himalayas are a place of astonishing ecological diversity, with microclimates including scrub forests, deciduous forests, evergreen forests, grasslands, savannahs, alpine meadows, and tundra. And in some of these microclimates, the goji berry was first harvested, consumed, and discovered to be a remarkable natural medicine by ancient people who resided in those mountains.

Himalayan traditional medicine is believed to have begun in the earliest days of human civilization. The Himalayans' healing methods are said to be the basis of today's traditional Tibetan and Chinese medical systems, as well as of India's ayurvedic system of medicine.

Not coincidentally, some of the people who live in and around this mountainous region are remarkably long-lived. Scientists have found that, among those living on the Plateau of the Yellow River in Inner Mongolia, life spans surpassing one hundred years are not nearly as uncommon as they are in the United States. A nearby part of Asia, the county of Pinghan in southwestern China, has one of the highest concentrations of centenarians on the planet. And the folks in the west Elbow Plateau and Pinghan—and in other parts of Asia where people commonly live very long and healthy lives—have one important thing in common: They eat goji berries. Lots and lots of goji berries.

Of course, the berries aren't the only factor. These people don't eat fast food or junk food. They are physically active and live in a place with clean air and water. Still, the role of the goji berry isn't one to ignore. As you'll see, these berries are extremely highly concentrated sources of nutrients. Throughout parts of Asia, the goji berry has been used in traditional medicine to promote longevity, to energize the body and build the blood, and to treat infertility.

I've had the privilege of attending the two-week festival held in China to honor the goji berry. This festival celebrates the role of the goji berry as food and medicine, and for its role in the region's folklore, literature, and history. For several decades, Asian scientists have tried to determine whether this food is all it has been cracked up to be by traditional healers. They've discovered that it is—and then some.

GOJI UNDER THE MICROSCOPE

The nutritional bounty of goji berries includes the following:

- More protein than whole wheat, with nineteen amino acids, including all eight of the essential aminos

- Twenty-one trace minerals, including germanium, which has been the subject of intense study because of its anticancer effects

- A wide spectrum of antioxidants, including vitamin C, vitamin E, flavonoids such as zeaxanthin, and various carotenoids such as beta-carotene

- B-complex vitamins

- Beta-sitosterol, a cholesterol-like compound found in plant foods that has anti-inflammatory, cholesterol-lowering effects, and has been used in natural medical research as a therapy for prostate enlargement and impotence

- Essential fatty acids

- A sesquiterpene called cyperone, which has beneficial effects for the circulatory system

- Physalin, a compound that is currently under investigation by ontological researchers because of its activity in vitro (in a test tube) against every major type of leukemia; physalin also has been found to promote the activity of cancer-killing natural killer (NK) cells in mouse experiments, and shows promise as a natural therapy for hepatitis

Pretty impressive lineup, right? There's more.

THE MASTER MOLECULES

The most exciting aspect of goji phytochemistry is its high content of bioactive polysaccharides, which I like to call "master molecules." These polysaccharides are complex carbohydrates bound to proteins. They are produced by some plants to defend against attack by parasites, viruses, fungi, bacteria, free radicals, and pollutants. They are also believed to help protect plants against cell mutations.

Goji grows best in rigorous conditions, with extremely cold winters and very hot summers. Like many other hardy plants, its very ability to thrive under extreme conditions is a clue to its medicinal potential for human beings. The more extreme the stresses under which a plant grows, the higher its content of these bioactive polysaccharides. When scientists used mass spectrometry to measure the content of these molecules in 9,031 berries from various locations, they were stunned by their nature and abundance in this particular fruit. Depending on the growing conditions, the content of these master molecules could vary significantly. Measuring their content in many goji samples—determining their "spectral signatures"—gave investigators the ability to determine which goji berries had the highest concentration of bioactive polysaccharides, and therefore which were most beneficial for human health.

HEALTH EFFECTS OF GOJI

Immunomodulator. Goji helps to reduce immune overreactivity—as seen in allergies and autoimmune conditions, such as psoriasis and Crohn's disease—and promote the immune system's responsiveness to pathogens, enhancing activity of T-cells and natural killer cells.

Anti-aging properties. Goji's antioxidant carotenoids and flavonoids, and its master molecules, collaborate to maintain cardiovascular health and improve the body's ability to cope with stress. In fact, goji is considered by many to be an adaptogen, which promotes natural, healthful physiological balance in all body systems.

Adaptogenic energizer. Asian athletes use this berry in the same way they might use other adaptogens, to increase endurance and strength, raise the fatigue threshold, and promote faster recovery after workouts. Research reveals that goji enhances the storage of glycogen, the stored form of carbohydrates. More stored glycogen translates into a quick, powerful burst of energy. What athlete wouldn't want that?

Anti-inflammatory properties. Goji consumption has been found to dramatically increase levels of an important anti-inflammatory enzyme, SOD (superoxide dismutase), in the body. SOD helps to control damage done by the superoxide free radical, which is implicated in conditions such as osteoarthritis.

Brain protector. A study by University of Hong Kong investigators found that goji could help protect against the cellular changes that lead to Alzheimer's disease: accumulation of toxic beta-amyloid in nerve cells. Through its antioxidant actions and another more complex cellular protective effect (too complex to explain here!), goji has been found to protect neurons against death due to the accumulation of beta-amyloid.

Heart healer. Antioxidants in goji help to prevent heart disease in several ways: (1) It reduces the oxidation of LDL (the so-called "bad" cholesterol) in the bloodstream by increasing SOD levels, and (2) through its antioxidant flavonoids and its master molecules, it improves endothelial function, enabling constricted blood vessels to relax and open.

Anticancer properties. Because goji contains the mineral germanium—in addition to its high concentration of antioxidant carotenoids and flavonoids and those fabulous master molecules—it protects against the onslaught of cancerous growth. Case reports from Asian practitioners who administered goji along with chemotherapy reveal that this food helps patients to better cope with toxic cancer therapies, and that patients' response rates to the drugs were vastly improved. Remissions achieved in patients who took goji were much longer than those achieved in patients who did not consume this food. And, finally, studies have shown that goji enhances the body's production of the cancer-killing agent interleukin-2 (IL-2). A recent study found that goji polysaccharides inhibited cancerous cell proliferation and induced apoptosis (cancer cell death) in an experimental model of liver cancer.

Antidepressant action. Asians don't call goji the "happy berry" without good reason. Legend has it that continued consumption of goji has one significant side effect: It makes you unable to stop smiling. This berry improves sleep and energy levels, and it's certainly worth trying if you are feeling emotionally low.

Antidiabetic, anti-obesity properties. Goji has long been used in Chinese medicine to treat diabetes. The master molecules have blood sugar–balancing effects. A recent series of studies in diabetic rats found that supplementing with goji helps protect against diabetic complications and may even promote improved insulin sensitivity. Obesity, a condition often related to diabetes, can also be ameliorated with daily consumption of goji. The master molecules aid in more efficient burning of food as energy (as opposed to its storage as fat). One study on human patients found that morning and afternoon helpings of goji promoted increased weight loss.

Improved sexual performance. Goji has long been revered as an aphrodisiac in Asian medicine. It has been found to boost testosterone levels and sexual stamina.

Recovery from periodontal surgery. One study found that goji polysaccharides, even in low doses, improved the attachment of new gum tissue following periodontal surgery.

Eye protector. Goji is a traditional Asian preventive medicine against loss of vision with aging. Recent research has shown that goji protects the ocular nerve against glaucoma in an experimental model.

MY RECOMMENDATIONS

Like any plant genus, *Lycium* encompasses dozens of plants, and many of them yield berries that can appropriately be called goji berries. But the truth is that only two types of *Lycium* berries have been studied as natural medicines: *Lycium barbarum* and *Lycium chinense*. The *L. chinense* is orange to light red, has many seeds, and is more tart—too sour to eat by itself. *Lycium chinense* is sometimes called Chinese wolfberry, matrimony vine, or Chinese boxthorn. *L. barbarum* is the ultimate goji berry—plump, red, and sweet, with very few seeds. It has the right spectral signature and nutrient density to qualify as the world's most nutrient-dense food, and it tastes wonderful.

The very best varieties, according to their spectral signatures, are said to be grown in one of two Chinese provinces—Ningxia and Xinjiang—or in the Himalayas.

Okay—convinced? If you're wavering, trust me—just try it. You'll never go back. What I recommend is daily consumption of goji juice. Try to drink one to four ounces (28–113g) of this ruby-red liquid per day. The juice you choose should be of the highest quality, with a spectral signature that matches that of Himalayan goji.

Like any natural medicine, goji doesn't instantly transform your body; it may take weeks or months for you to feel a difference. Drink it in good health!

21

Adding Years to Your Life and Life to Your Years

Richard A. Passwater, PhD

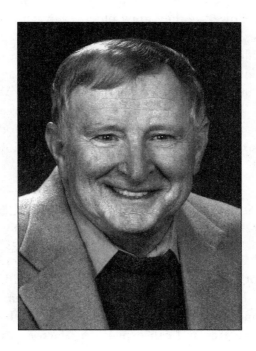

Richard Passwater, a research biochemist and one of the world's lead-ing experts on selenium, has written numerous books and magazine articles on nutrition, including the best-selling *Supernutrition: Mega-vitamin Revolution*. He also writes a monthly column for *Whole Foods* magazine. Website: www.drpasswater.com

Yes, it is not only possible to add fifteen to twenty years of healthy life to your years—but practical to do so as well. The question in your mind now may be, "Well, if this is indeed practical, how do I do it?" This is a question that I have often been asked since I presented my integrated theory of aging to the Gerontological Society in Toronto in October 1970, and I will summarize my research findings, plus the findings of other gerontolgists in terms of lifestyle and nutrition here.

I wasn't studying the aging process because I wanted to live longer. As both an athlete and a scientist, I wanted to know why athletes became a little slower as they grew older, even if they ate the most nutritious foods and exercised hard. Why couldn't the well-tuned body of the athlete remain at peak performance with the best nourishment and training? What changes occur with age and why?

Still today, I am not just interested in living longer. What is important to me is to live *better* longer. The goal is to increase the quality of life as well as the length of life. We want to add more years to our lives, but we also want to add more life to our years. Slowing the aging process is all about living better and longer.

THERE'S MORE TO LIVING BETTER LONGER THAN THE GENES YOU'RE BORN WITH!

What practical steps can you take to live better longer? Most people realize that a lot of our health and longevity starts with the genes we are born with. However, few people realize that our nourishment, environment, and lifestyle greatly affect our genes. Today, scientists understand this better and can explain this factor in terms of gene expression. Having certain gene variations is one thing, but turning the genes off or on is something else. The important thing is that you have more control over your genes than scientists used to think and that there are indeed practical things you can do to turn on your good genes and turn off your bad genes.

Before we learned how nutrients interact with our genes to turn them on and off, research efforts were aimed primarily at reducing the damage that causes aging. Then we moved on to learning how to repair this damage. In 1991, it was discovered that some of the same nutrients that protect the body against the damage that leads to aging also have a functional role in turning many genes on and off.

PROVEN COMMON-SENSE LONGEVITY PRACTICES

I will give you a short list of what scientific studies have shown are some of the most practical things you can do to help you live better longer. Some of the advice is not new: It's basically common sense and the moderation that Mom taught us, but now there is also scientific validation for those practices as well. Some of my points are lifestyle factors, but most are nutritional. The strategy is to slow the damage to essential body components with antioxidant nutrients, to increase the rate of repair of these damaged components, and to selectively turn on good genes and turn off bad genes. In the future, we will simply be able to reconstruct our genes so as to have only good genes.

Whatever your genes, you can take steps to live a longer, healthier life. Common findings among those who study centenarians include the following:

- Live a healthy life. Don't smoke. Drink only in moderation. Wear your seat belt.

- Watch the calories! Eat a diet rich in fruits and vegetables, low in animal and saturated fat.

- Be active! At the minimum, exercise thirty minutes a day, three times a week. Include cardiovascular exercise and strength training in your workout regimen.

- Keep a positive attitude! Stay engaged in life. Make new friends and keep up with old friends. If you can, volunteer at a local hospital or charity.

- Challenge your brain. Solve puzzles and/or learn new skills.

I will extend these general observations with some of my own later in the conclusion.

DAMAGE THAT ACCELERATES AGING

For the past forty years, I have focused my research on preventing damage in the body that leads to aging. My integrated theory of aging is based primarily on laboratory animal research I conducted in the 1960s and 1970s. Today my research efforts are geared toward combating aging and cancer.

My research has not been directed at the primary factor of aging that determines the human life span as a species, but at the secondary factor of aging that determines how long we live within our species limit. In other words, it has not been aimed at the process that determines that a mouse will live for a couple of years, a dog for about 15 years and a tortoise over 100. Instead, it has been aimed at helping more of us reach our current human life span of about 115 years and, more importantly, live those extra years in excellent health! So my research has been focusing on slowing the aging process.

After my presentation to the Gerontological Society in 1970, I published my results showing that certain synergistic combinations of nutrients extended the average life span of laboratory mice by 20–30 percent and the maximum life span by 5–10 percent. The greater increase in average life span as compared to maximum life span suggested that diseases like cancer were being affected as well as aging. A series of laboratory animal experiments quickly confirmed that this was the case.

There is no one physical or mental condition directly attributed simply to the passage of time. It is not the passage of time that ages us; it is the accumulation of deleterious chemical events that deteriorates our bodies into the condition we call aging. What, then, is aging?

Aging is the process that reduces the number of healthy cells in the body. The most striking factor in the aging process is the body's loss of reserve, due to the decreasing number of cells in each organ. The mass of healthy active cells in each organ declines as a person ages; thus, the organ's function is diminished. Simply stated, the aging process is the body's loss of ability to respond to a challenge to its status quo (homeostasis).

Now the question becomes this: What causes this loss of reserve? Much of the damage that destroys healthy cells results from reactive compounds that are formed as by-products during the normal chemical reactions of the life process. These reactive by-products are called free radicals and reactive oxygen species. It is not important to understand how they work, just to recognize that they are there and they are detrimental to health.

Free radical reactions result in the body's loss of active cells. The cumulative effect of billions of cellular free radical reactions is the loss of cells. This happens in several ways.

1. Free radical damage to the cell membranes can impair the cell's ability to transport nutrients into the cell and the cell dies without replacing itself.

2. Free radical damage to cell membranes can impair the cell's ability to transport waste products out of the cell; thus, the cell can drown in its own waste. The result is that the cell can die without replacing itself.

3. Free radicals can damage the cell's DNA so that, instead of the cell being replaced by another healthy daughter cell, the cell is replaced with a mutant that doesn't function correctly.

4. Free radicals can damage the lysosomal sac and release deadly lysosomes, which are enzymes that destroy other cell components. This leaves the cell devoid of working parts and it cannot be replaced. The cell becomes a clunker and the body becomes one cell older.

5. Free radicals can fuse proteins together so they do not function properly. This can damage a cell so that it does not perform and does not reproduce a healthy replacement.

6. Free radical reactions form by-products, such as the age pigment lipofuscin or advanced glycosolated end products. These residues accumulate over time and interfere with cell function.

The result of many of the free radical reactions is that the number of active cells in the body decrease.

Forming the body's defense against free radicals are compounds that neutralize them by giving up electrons to the radicals. Such compounds are called antioxidants. Dietary antioxidants are very important to our body's defense against these harmful compounds. There are thousands of nutritional antioxidants that can be found in food. Some antioxidant nutrients are especially important and are provided as dietary supplements. These are included in my recommendations in the Conclusion.

CONCLUSION

I am a biochemist and I deal exclusively with proven facts about chemicals, electron cloud distributions, chemical pathways, and chemical reactions. That said, please understand that some chemical reactions are actually thought processes that affect other chemical reactions. The mind and body are chemically interrelated and inseparable. Thoughts affect body chemistry.

My research suggests to me that the most important aspect of living better longer is to develop happiness and peace! Notice that I used the word *develop*, not *find*. The mind can be trained to be happy and peaceful. This reduces stress and improves brain chemistry, which, in turn, improves body chemistry.

Do you have a happy mind? How do you develop a happy mind if you don't have one? Here's my test to see if you have a happy mind. Answer immediately without thinking. On a scale of 1 to 10, with 10 being the highest rating, where do you rate your level of happiness? If you immediately answer 9 or 10, you probably have a very happy mind. If you had to think about it, or rated your level below 9, you need to work on it to optimize your longevity potential.

One thing is certain about having a happy mind. It has nothing at all to do with materialism. There are more poor people in poor countries happier than materialistically "well-off" people in wealthy countries. You can learn to be happy. If you already have a happy mind, devote about fifteen minutes each day to a meditation period in which you think only happy thoughts and count your blessings. No negative thoughts allowed. If you haven't developed a happy mind yet, make this happiness meditation period a daily half-hour. Within two weeks, your mind will be transformed and your body chemistry improved. Stress effects will also diminish. The manner in which you handle your stress will also improve. You may not be able to remove the cause of stress, but you can defeat stress by not allowing the cause to ruin your body chemistry. Happiness is the stress antidote and happiness is effective rather than "forced" or natural.

Next in importance is to eat and drink in moderation. Fear no food, but understand appropriate amounts. Eat foods produced by nature, or close to nature, rather than foods made in factories with mostly processed ingredients. Use table salt sparingly. It's OK to have an occasional piece of cake to celebrate, but a diet overloaded with junk food is deadly. Studies show that most people live longer having one alcoholic drink a day than those who abstain or overindulge. One way to achieve moderation in your diet is to include variety. Eating some of many different foods is better than eating a lot of any one food.

After the foundation of a happy mind and a healthy diet is established, then the body can be strengthened by dietary supplements. Some supplements can effect pronounced additional improvement in living better longer. However, supplements will not be as effective if the body is not adequately nourished by a good diet in the first place.

Based on my own research, plus an evaluation of the scientific literature, I am convinced that the following daily supplement program will help people live better longer.

- A good multivitamin/multimineral
- Vitamin C: 2,000–4,000 mg (divided doses)
- Pycnogenol: 50–100 mg
- Coenzyme Q_{10}: 30–100 mg
- Alpha-lipoic acid: 25–100 mg (divided doses)
- Acetyl-l-carnitine (or other amino carnitine): 500 mg
- Resveratrol: 500 mg (or more)
- Fish oil or DHA: 1,000–3,000 mg (divided doses)
- Phosphatidylserine: 500 mg
- Magnesium: 400 mg
- Selenium: 200 mcg
- Vitamin D_2: 500 IU

- Vitamin K$_2$: 50 mg

- L-arginine: 500 mg

- Silicon: 10–25 mg

Finally, adopt a healthy lifestyle of not smoking, being active, and practicing moderation in drinking. Socialize and volunteer to help others. Your life will become better immediately and you will live better longer. Good luck.

22

Diabesity

Fred Pescatore, MD, MPH, CCN

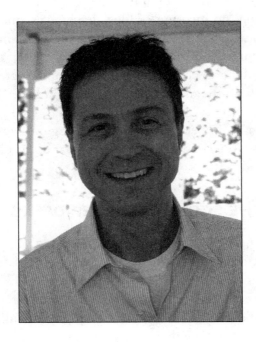

Fred Pescatore is one of the key spokespersons for healthy living. His latest *New York Times* best-sellers, *The Hamptons Diet* and *The Hamptons Diet Cookbook,* combine the Mediterranean lifestyle with the palates of Americans, emphasizing a whole-foods approach to health and weight management. He lectures around the world, is the host of a weekly radio broadcast, and has been seen on such shows as *Today, The View, AM Canada,* and many others. Address: 369 Lexington Avenue—19th Floor, New York, NY 10017. Tel: 212-779-2944. Website: www.drpescatore.com

While many people have been clamoring to stake a claim to this very poignant and real problem facing America today, I first heard the term *diabesity* from the lips of one of the founding fathers of nutritional medicine today, Robert C. Atkins, MD. He was the first person that I can ever remember putting these two health issues together so eloquently. At the time, some fourteen years ago, I was the associate medical director for his medical clinic in New York City.

This was my first real glimpse into the arena that eating affects your health. In medical school, that concept was not even taught. People got sick, and you prescribed a pill to make them better. There was no talk of prevention, no mention of lifestyle changes, and certainly no classes taught on clinical nutrition. By beginning my medical career at the Atkins Center, I saw people taking charge of their health for the first time, not willing to chalk things up to "I'm just getting old," and getting well without the use of potentially harmful prescription medications. It opened my eyes and, in this short essay, I am going to share with you how to avoid becoming one of the legions who fall prey to the sad Standard American Diet, and how to prevent obesity and all its devastating side effects.

THE SCOPE OF THE EPIDEMIC

When it comes to diabetes and obesity, it is certainly possible to have one without the other; that is to say, you can be obese and not have diabetes and you can be diabetic and certainly not be obese. But the epidemic we face today and the ballooning health care costs associated with both diabetes and obesity are very closely linked.

Obesity is responsible, either directly or indirectly, for four of the top ten leading causes of death in the United States: heart disease, cancer, stroke, and diabetes. Obesity affects one in three Americans and one in four children. If this continues, everyone in the United States will be obese or overweight by the year 2025. Obesity costs one in five health care dollars spent—a staggering sum and one we cannot afford.

Diabetes, on the other hand, is known to affect about 20 million Americans and an estimated 20 million more are undiagnosed diabetics. So almost half the people who have the disease don't even know they have it. In fact, I screen all my patients for diabetes and roughly 25 percent of them aren't aware that they are affected. And I have a practice that is nutrition-oriented. During a clinical trial I ran in India, over 70 percent of the patients we screened were diabetic and didn't know it. I suggest you get tested immediately.

Diabetes is the leading cause of blindness and amputation in the United States. It can lead to high blood pressure, kidney disease, gangrene, and impotence, to name just a few of the devastating effects it can have on your body. We have been lulled into the false impression that it is a disease that we can live with. That is true on one level, but it is basically an illness that kills you slowly every day.

HOW DO THE TWO CONNECT?

Obesity is the leading health risk factor for contracting diabetes. There are two distinct types of diabetes—types 1 and 2. In the past, type 1 was considered juvenile diabetes, because that is when you were diagnosed with it; type 2 was considered adult-onset. We can no longer use those classifications because so many children are being diagnosed with type 2 diabetes. This is the type where the body produces insulin but is unable to use it. You may have heard this referred to as insulin resistance or syndrome X. When I was in medical school not too long ago, it was unheard of to diagnose children with type 2 diabetes. Now, the youngest person to be diagnosed with this condition was seven years old and the numbers are growing exponentially each year.

So we are quite literally eating ourselves to death. And we are encouraging our children to do the same. When you eat, your pancreas has to secrete a hormone called insulin in order to bring your blood sugar down. This is a normal response to eating. When you eat too many simple carbohydrates or too much sugar as your abundant fuel source, which so many people do, this puts a strain on the delicate balance between insulin secretion, the hormone receptors, and your body's ability to bring blood sugar back down to the normal range.

Over time, this eventually leads to insulin resistance, which simply means that your body has to produce more insulin to do the same job it once did. Your receptors are losing their ability to process the insulin efficiently. This is analogous to a drug abuser who needs ever-increasing amounts of the drug to get the same effect he enjoyed when he first started abusing. Congratulations—you are now on the road to diabetes.

At some point, this system will break down as you continue to consume lots of processed foods, pasta, white bread, cake, sugar, pretzels, soda (or liquid corn, as I like to call it), and fruit juice. And for those of you who think that fruit juice is a natural sugar and there couldn't possibly be anything wrong with that, let's just tackle that myth head-on. Sugar is sugar is sugar, no matter how it is disguised. Sugar, by its very definition is a natural product—it grows from the ground and is processed into many different food forms. Honey, molasses, and anything that ends in -ose and -ol are all forms of sugar. It is all metabolized by the body in the same exact way.

In fact, there have been numerous clinical studies that have shown us that children who drink more fruit juice are at higher risk of contracting type 2 diabetes than those who drink far less. The same holds true for soda, which is proving to be even less healthy, not because of the chemicals it contains but because it is sweetened with high-fructose corn syrup—a sugar substitute that tends to raise blood sugar even faster than ordinary sugar.

THE ROAD TO RECOVERY

At last we come to the easy part of the essay. The association between diabetes, obesity, and health is quite complex, and modern medical science is only beginning to unravel all the multiple associations; however, we are coming to understand and study ways in which we can help ourselves overcome this problem. We ate ourselves into the problem and we can eat ourselves out of the problem. Unfortunately, we have a health care system that is solely based on treating illness, not preventing it, so the battle is just beginning.

The program I recommend to patients and the programs I have outlined in my books, obviously fine-tuned through the years as we learn fresh food science, can be summed up in a few sentences. We need to eat more like our ancestors and more like our compatriots in the Mediterranean lands. Lean proteins, such as fish, pork, and some red meat; vegetables, nuts, seeds, healthy fats and oils, whole grains (not processed ones), beans, legumes, and fruits—these are the foods we should eat. Anything else is inconsistent with our diet and goes against nature. And, if these foods can be fresh, local, seasonal, and organic, even better.

We have become programmed to believe that packaged, processed, and fast foods (no matter how healthy they seem) are good for us. And if not good for us, at least they are a quick alternative. Real food is the key to a long life.

Each meal should consist of a protein—beef, chicken, turkey, pork, eggs, and so on—along with vegetables. Here is another common pitfall most of us make. Vegetables are not peas (they are a legume), corn (a starch), and potatoes (another starch). Those are the most common vegetables Americans consume, and none of them have much to do with vegetables.

Don't be afraid to eat nuts, as many of them are filled with heart-healthy fats, such as omega-3 fatty acids or, in the case of macadamia nuts, the heart-healthiest, omega-9 fat. We have been led down a false road into thinking that all fats are unhealthy. They aren't; however, that is the basis for another essay entirely. Just keep in mind that canola oil is unhealthy and *never* use it for any purpose. Olive oil is great for cold uses but never heat it, and use a high-heat oil that is loaded with monounsaturated fats, such as macadamia nut, avocado, or hazelnut oil for cooking purposes.

Beans, legumes, and whole grains have their place in our diets. However, in my experience, I recommend these as side dishes and not main courses, so eat them sparingly but don't be afraid of them. In my practice, I tend to recommend beans and legumes over grains.

Lastly, as for fruits, I tend to recommend the lower-sugar fruits, which are basically anything other than tropical fruits like bananas (yes, America's number one fruit—get potassium from a nutritional supplement instead), pineapples, mangoes, and the like. Stick to the lower-sugar fruits, such as berries and melons—and please consume seasonal fruits if you can.

There can be no simpler diet—eat real foods, minimally processed and optimally nutritious.

HELPFUL HINTS

There is no magic to eating healthy—just dedication. We need to kick our fast food habits. We need to learn how to cook again. We need to stop ordering in. In the generation from when I was a kid to now, the kitchen has become one of the largest rooms in a new home and one of the least used. Cooking food can take as little time as waiting for the delivery. Learning a few very basic recipes can save your life.

Go to your local grocery store and learn where the healthier foods are. Learn to cook ahead of time so you are never in a rush or never in a hunger-panicked situation where there is nothing to eat that is remotely healthy. Stop buying unhealthy foods and keeping them in the house for guests, the kids, your spouse, company. They do not need to be there and won't get eaten if they are unavailable.

I often prepare a weeks' worth of breakfasts on a Sunday so they can easily be reheated as I am rushing out the door. Packing lunches, if they are prepared ahead of time can be a snap. Just learn to prepare ahead and eat defensively. In other words, don't wait until you are starving to decide what to eat and never go grocery shopping on an empty stomach.

I know a lot of what I have just said is common sense. But, truth be told, eating in a healthy way to prevent heart disease, diabetes, and many common health ailments is very common wisdom and, yes, our parents and grandparents were right in many respects when it comes to food. We are what we eat and therefore, eating should not be secondary. Eating should be a primary concern and something we teach our kids first and foremost.

The ability to put an end to the diabesity epidemic and keep yourself away from its clutches is within your grasp. Armed with this information, I challenge you to make your next grocery store trip a healthy experience and not one just to get sustenance. Learn to like what is healthy for you and don't get caught up in the food industrial complex hype. Less is the new more.

23

Why and How to
'Doctor Yourself'

Andrew W. Saul

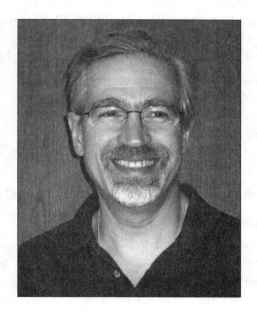

Andrew W. Saul, who has over thirty years' experience in natural health education, has taught nutrition, health science, and cell biology at the college level for nine years. Saul is the winner of three New York State teacher fellowships, the Citizens for Health Outstanding Health Freedom Activist Award, and was named one of seven natural health pioneers by *Psychology Today* magazine. He is editor of the *Orthomolecular Medicine News Service,* and assistant editor of the *Journal of Orthomolecular Medicine*. Saul is the author of the popular books *Doctor Yourself: Natural Healing That Works* and *Fire Your Doctor! How to Be Independently Healthy*. Address: 141 Main Street, Brockport, New York 14420. Website: www.doctoryourself.com

Be careful in reading health books.
You may die of a misprint.

—MARK TWAIN

If you want something done right, you have to do it yourself. This especially includes your health care. That is why I am what I call a "health homesteader." For me, it became personal when, over thirty years ago, my firstborn was placed in my arms. As a newly minted father, the first thing I had to do was take my newborn out of the hospital immediately. They were feeding the baby formula and he was getting feverish. At home, with vitamins and breast milk, he thrived. A well baby checkup resulted in a vaccination that made a goose-egg-sized lump at the injection site and gave the baby a high fever. The pediatrician seemed to know no more than the hospital. Now I was working without a net: I had to learn—and fast. In the end, I was able to raise my children all the way to college without a single dose of any antibiotic. Yes, we had family doctors, whom we never went to. So since 1976, I have been teaching people how to get well and stay well.

ORTHOMOLECULAR NUTRITION

There are various paths to health. Taking appropriately high doses of vitamins and other needed nutrients is the great superhighway. May I add that I have no financial connection whatsoever with the health products industry. Vitamins, in appropriately high doses, are both preventive and therapeutic. If you have a cold, or feel one coming on, and you take a gram (1,000 mg) of vitamin C every five minutes, you will feel better in hours. Loose stool indicates saturation. My jingle is, "Take enough C to be symptom free, whatever that amount might be." If you are stressed or anxious, take a few hundred milligrams of niacin (B_3) and you will feel better in minutes. You may experience a harmless warm flush. But to learn more, to determine you own best doses, you need to do what I did: Read. To take it to the next level, I suggest you read everything you can by Robert F. Cathcart III, MD; Frederick R. Klenner, MD; and Abram Hoffer, MD, PhD (who contributed an essay to this collection). These are three of the great orthomolecular (nutritional) physicians. My most concise advice is this: Do what works and copy the doctors who get results. Perhaps that is why you are reading this book right now.

Part of the appeal of aggressive nutritional supplementation is that taking tablets is easier than changing your lifestyle. Supplement therapy is very effective and also very safe. U.S. poison control statistics show that there is not even one death per year from vitamin supplementation. On the other hand, research indicates that inadequate nutrition annually kills literally millions, and is probably the single largest cause of death there is. All, and I mean *all*, of the big killer diseases are primarily caused by bad diet. Lousy nutrition never cured anything; optimum nutrition has. See for yourself: You can read the full archive of the peer-reviewed *Journal of Orthomolecular Medicine* for free at http://orthomolecular.org/library/jom or http://www.ortho med.org/jom/jom.html.

In case you thought you'd get out of this with a few tablets, well, think again. I also urge diet and lifestyle change, and personally practice what I am here recommending to you. At age fifty-three, I am in better shape than when I was in college. OK, that was the far-out early '70s, but still. Today I can shovel snow literally by the ton (there is a lot of that in Brockport, New York), walk for miles, touch my knuckles to the floor, do a thousand crunches, and sleep well.

I advocate a near-vegetarian diet. Note the word *near*. I am not a vegetarian, although I respect and even advocate vegetarianism for those who feel best with it. I personally choose to include eggs, seafood, and cultured dairy products in my diet. In moderation, these foods are good for you, and I raised my children accordingly. I eat meat three or four times a week, usually less. But the real focus should be a plant-based diet. Need to lose a few pounds? This will do it. You will automatically reach your right weight with a plant-based diet. Weigh in once a week and see. The high-fiber content of near-veggie fare will also make you feel better in other ways in the bathroom, and also help prevent cardiovascular disease and cancer. One of the dangers of meat-eating is that meat has zero fiber. Modest meat-eating is greatly mitigated by having the rest of your diet high-fiber and plant-based. Whole grains and legumes (peas, beans, lentils) are terrific foods, versatile and cheap. Many of the negative aspects of meat and dairy relate to excess consumption and excess factory processing. Cold cuts laced with chemical additives, and the white water served up as milk nowadays should be the first to vanish from your table. Yogurt and aged cheeses have my vote, but since I'm a former dairyman, you'd expect that. May I add that we should also weigh the lives of the critters we kill. If all of us decreased our meat intake by only 10 percent, we'd save the lives of over 1 billion animals each year. Think about it: If you currently eat some meat at practically every meal, just two meatless meals a week gives you that 10 percent reduction.

It is very important to maintain a low-sugar diet. Whatever may be ailing you, sugar is sure to make it worse. The best writers on this subject are Drs. T. L. Cleave, Lendon H. Smith, and Abram Hoffer. Yes, we need to consciously, daily, work to avoid sugar. It isn't easy, is it? If you are going to have some anyway, as most folks do including me, here's some absolution: Some sugar is far better that any artificial sweeteners. OK, enough of that. Now here's what to do:

1. Take a B-complex vitamin tablet, some chromium, lots of vitamin C, and some extra niacin whenever you eat sugar. It will greatly help to even out both your mood and your blood sugar levels.

2. Eat sweet stuff only if you are about to exercise and burn it off before your body stores it as fat.

While moderation is often the healthiest policy, there are some clear-cut absolute no-nos.

1. No junk food! This automatically and instantly reduces your intake of salt, fat, and chemical food additives. Check your kitchen sink and kitchen garbage can every day. Greasy dishes and convenience-food wrappers mean trouble. A big vegetable-peeling pile composting in the backyard means success.

2. No artificial colors! Why eat paint? For that, come back from the hardware store with a spoon instead of a brush. Of all the many food additives, colors are the worst. Check the Internet to see what the Feingold Association has to say about this.

3. No over-the-counter medicines! Use vitamins instead. As Carl C. Pfeiffer said, there is a natural alternative to every drug. In most cases, this goes for prescription drugs as well. Linus Pauling put it

best when he suggested that every drug should have a printed label, warning: "Keep this medicine out of reach of everyone! Use vitamin C instead."

OTHER RECOMMENDATIONS

It is well worth your while to learn some basic homeopathy; John Henry Clarke's *Prescriber* is still the best single volume to help you. If you learn a remedy per week, that's fifty in a year with a two-week vacation. You can start with arnica, excellent for strains and sprains. In raising a family, I constantly used the twelve Schuessler cell minerals (Kali Phos for irritability; Calc Phos for teething).

Question immunizations. At the very least, give your children boatloads of vitamin C before they get the needle. Delay immunizations to at least age two. Vitamin supplemented, unprocessed-food-fed children are healthier, shots or no shots.

Drink lots of water, but try to avoid fluoridated water. The lifetime benefit of drinking fluoridated water amounts to one-half of one filling less per person. On the other hand, fluoride is harmful at far lower levels than the EPA-permitted four parts per million. The more you read on this, the clearer it will all be. The Internet, not your dentist, is your best bet for more information.

Avoid doctors and hospitals. I last saw my GP over twelve years ago. Health self-reliance is not about refusing needed medical care; it is about putting yourself in a position of not needing medical care.

Garden. It is good for body and soul, and organic food can't be cheaper. No land? When in doubt, sprout. Sprouted seeds have more nutrition. Wheat and lentils are dirt cheap, and sprout in any old jar in two days. It's easy to toss them into a salad or sandwich.

If you feel ill, fast first. The old misquoted phrase should read, "Starve a cold lest you feed a fever." The first thing a sick animal does is go off its food. Right. More comfortable than water fasting is a temporary diet of raw vegetable juices only. As my uncle would say, it is "good for what ails you."

Exercise. The best exercise for you is the one that you will actually do. Regular practice of yoga provides gentle and yet remarkably thorough exercise. Tension, stress, and many a back problem disappear.

Eliminate bad habits. Mark Twain tells of a doctor at the bedside of a very sick, elderly lady. The doctor told her that she must stop drinking, cussing, and smoking. The lady said that she'd never done any of those things in her entire life. The doctor responded, "Well, that's your problem, then. You've neglected your habits." Twain added: "She was like a sinking ship with no freight to throw overboard." But seriously, if you smoke, drink, take drugs, or bungee-jump with a frayed cord, you are, as my mother always said, just looking for trouble. Taking high doses of vitamin C will help you break the smoking habit; ditto for drugs. Frequent large doses of the B-complex vitamins will help you stop drinking.

Reduce stress. I have practiced Transcendental Meditation for thirty years, and I have only good to say about it. Other forms of meditation, many of which I have also tried, are also very valuable. Pick one and do it. Ahh, it works. And be sure to hit the hay early. I like to be asleep by 10 p.m. Ben Franklin was right about that early-to-bed bit.

SUPPLEMENTS I TAKE EACH DAY
TO PREVENT ILLNESS

- Vitamin C: 15,000–20,000 mg, divided up into (approximately hourly) doses
- Vitamin E (natural mixed tocopherols): 600–800 IU
- Lecithin: 1–2 tablespoons (a good and cheap source of inositol, choline, and essential fatty acids)
- Vitamin D: 1,500 IU
- Fish oil: 2,000 mg (360 mg EPA; 240 mg DHA)
- Zinc: 100 mg
- Magnesium: 300–400 mg, with some calcium
- Chromium: 200–400 mcg

If you don't see a specific nutrient listed above, such as B-complex vitamins or selenium, it's in the three high-potency multivitamins that

I take, one with every meal. I also take some mealtime multiple digestive enzyme tablets. I estimate that my supplements cost me far less than a buck a day. In my opinion, that is the best $365-per-year health insurance you can buy.

So I'm a health nut, right? But if you are not a health nut, then what kind of a nut are you? For those who choose not to take care of themselves, perhaps this is the time to say that universal health coverage is not the answer. Perhaps universal funeral coverage would be more appropriate. The bottom line is this: Compared to death, and not seeing your great-grandchildren, the odds greatly favor being a health nut. And it feels so good! Of course, I'll let you know for sure in another fifty-three years. Orthomolecular nutrition has served me well so far. I think it will help you, too. Remember: No cell in the human body is made from a drug. Not one. They are all made from what you eat. And what you eat—or won't eat—is totally within your control.

24

The Pillars of My Health— and Yours

Stephen T. Sinatra, MD, FACC, CNS

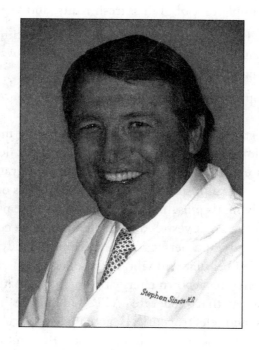

Stephen Sinatra, a nutritionally oriented cardiologist, was one of the first American cardiologists to adopt the clinical use of vitaminlike co-enzyme Q_{10} in the treatment of heart disease. His books include *Reverse Heart Disease Now* and *The Sinatra Solution: Metabolic Cardiology.* Address: The Optimum Health Building, 257 East Center Street, Manchester, CT 06040. Tel: 860-647-9729. Fax: 860-643-2531. Website: www. opthealth.com

As a physician for thirty-five years, I have learned a lot about healthy and graceful aging and the way to achieve it are really basic. Long ago I was impressed by the research of a Russian gerontologist who reported his findings in *National Geographic*. He examined twenty thousand healthy people aged 80 and above, many of whom were over 100. Here are the key factors that he found most of them had in common:

- They worked outside, weather permitting, getting sunlight, fresh air, and physical activity.

- They ate a simple diet of grains, fresh fruits, and vegetables.

- They enjoyed good relationships, rich in love, intimacy, and support. From cuddling and kissing to intercourse, it was the holding and the intimacy that meant the most to them.

- They were optimistic about life.

I try to go a step beyond his perspective by placing my cardiologist "spin" on his simple and sage observations. I've spent decades analyzing the body's electrical potential in electrocardiograms (ECGs or EKGs), watching its ultrasonic synchronous vibrations on echocardiograms, and studying its pulsating structures in invasive procedures like angiography of the great vessels and chambers. I have come to appreciate the complexity and perfection of the human body, and also the key importance of cellular and vibrational energy.

Every cell generates its own energy through enzymatic reactions in the mitochondria that generate ATP (adenosine triphosphate). Nutraceuticals and electroceuticals actually support this function when the body is in a state of optimum health. But, in order to understand pathology and illness, we need to focus on the damage that happens to the repair loops in each cell.

The health of the cell is negatively impacted by bodily trauma, emotional trauma, environmental toxins, pharmaceutical drugs, and electrical pollution. When the cells are bombarded with one or more of these agents, a departure from their healthy electrical potential and synchronous vibration occurs.

It is my firm belief that the reason we become ill—whether it be heart disease or any other condition—has more to do with the jeopardized integrity of the cellular membrane of each and every cell than anything else. Whatever the target organ(s), when the cell membrane is threatened, normal functioning is impaired. Simply stated, a healthy, semipermeable cell wall (membrane) allows nutrients in and toxins out.

To be healthy, the cell's membrane must be able to "breathe" as it ushers in the nutrients that support its metabolism and safely transports out the waste products of those chemical reactions to be excreted. In other words, the cellular membrane must be able to "inhale" oxygen, water, glucose, nutrients, hormones, and so forth and "exhale" waste and toxic by-products.

When the integrity of the cell membrane is impaired, microbial production increases. The invasion of microbes initiates and provokes degenerative processes that eventually cause insidious and relentless inflammation, a cycle that, left unchecked, continuously damages the cell. The key to intercepting this process is to sustain cellular energy.

Diseased cells, particularly cancerous ones, function at far lower cellular energy levels than healthy ones. Cells functioning at higher energy (i.e., ATP) levels have intact repair loops that "repair" themselves. So, energy preservation is key to optimum health and is integral to both a preventive and recovery approach to health maintenance.

There are many valid theories about the causes of aging, each of which champions a different approach for anti-aging strategies:

- the neuroendocrine theory (growth hormone)
- the endocrine theory (hormonal replacement)
- the free radical theory (oxidative stress)
- the mitochondrial theory (ATP)

This last (mitochondrial) makes the most sense to me. Why?

Every cell has the same basic structures, in addition to being specialized. Unlike well-armored nuclear DNA (the genetic material in the nucleus of the cell), mitochondrial DNA have no defense mechanisms. The mitochondria—nicknamed the "powerhouses of the cell"—generate the chemical energy (ATP) that is transferred to mechanical energy. In the heart muscle cell, that means managing cellular respiration, contracting and relaxing, conducting impulses, and so on.

In the process of mitochondrial respiration and the genesis of ATP, not all the oxygen is converted to carbon dioxide and water. Three to 5 percent of the oxygen generated results in breakdown products called free radicals. Because mitochondrial DNA has no defense mechanisms, it is vulnerable to these unstable, unpaired electrons. So it is absolutely essential to repair and support vulnerable mitochondrial function from relentless free radical stress.

In cardiology, solving the heart's energy crisis is essential to optimizing cardiovascular function. For decades, heart disease prevention has inadvertently been focused on lowering lipids (cholesterol) in an effort to prevent or slow coronary artery disease. Rather, it behooves us to shift the focus to the mitochondria and employ nutritional strategies targeting improved ATP synthesis and, therefore, heart function. So keep this biochemical/metabolic model in mind, and specifically focus on the concept of cellular energy and ATP production as I highlight for you the five pillars for health and longevity.

PILLAR I: NONINFLAMMATORY, NON–INSULIN-PROVOKING DIET

One of the best ways to nurture your cellular membranes is to bathe them with things they don't have to defend themselves against. Avoid produce exposed to toxic chemicals, particularly pesticides (which are proven to be carcinogenic), synthetic fertilizers, human waste, sewage sludge. Don't eat vegetables with the waxy coatings found on conventionally grown varieties to give them more eye appeal. Organic or free-range meats are not laced with hormones, insecticides, pesticides.

In addition to eating fresh organic fruits and vegetables, follow a diet that doesn't get your blood sugar spiking (we call this a non–insulin-provoking diet plan). Sugar ages you and causes diabetes.

All simple sugars, especially high-fructose corn syrup, should be avoided; they are powerful triggers of the inflammation that causes damage to cellular repair loops. Insulin, particularly in high concentration, is a powerful promoter of inflammation. To keep insulin levels low and on an even keel, eat some healthy protein at every meal, limit sugars, avoid caffeine, and keep high-glycemic carbohydrates to a minimum.

I suggest a dietary plan that incorporates the following:

- low-glycemic carbohydrates, like lentils, chickpeas, and broccoli
- healthy fats, especially omega-3s and monounsaturated fats
- high-quality organic proteins, like wild Alaskan salmon, organic nuts, free-range meats and free-range DHA-fortified eggs.
- plenty of clean drinking water (more on this later)

I also encourage you to eliminate trans fats from your diet and use polyunsaturated fats sparingly. The omission of trans-fatty acids protects cellular membranes, as well as adrenal glands, from the assaults of the free radicals they generate.

My Top 12 Healing Foods

All foods listed below are organic, natural, wild, or free range. These are the foods I eat in my everyday life.

1. Avocado—Contains lots of vitamin E, glutathione, and healthy monounsaturated fat.

2. Onions—Contain many compounds (flavonoids and quercetin) that enhance the immune system and improve prostate health.

3. Asparagus—Loaded with folic acid, vitamin C, and glutathione.

4. Spinach—Popeye was right. Rich in lutein, which helps prevent macular degeneration and is instrumental in both lung and heart health. An excellent source of calcium.

5. Wild blueberries—Contain flavonoids that improve the macula and retina of the eye and also help brain function.

6. Pomegranate juice—Contains powerful antioxidants, shown to assist in plaque regression.

7. Free-range buffalo—An outstanding source of protein with minimal saturated fat. No hormones, antibiotics, or chemicals.

Grass-fed buffalo also contain the fatty acids your body needs—omega-3s.

8. Wild Alaskan salmon—Rich in omega-3s and the vital carotenoid astaxanthin that helps prevent damaging oxidation in the body. It is seventeen times more powerful than pycnogenol and fifty times more powerful than vitamin E.

9. Broccoli—Full of sulfur compounds that assist in detoxifying the body, including anticancer compounds like sulforaphane and indole-3-carbinol.

10. Almonds—Contain monounsaturated fat, plus precious gamma tocopherol, a vital nutrient that neutralizes perioxynitrite, a dangerous free radical that destroys cellular endothelial membranes.

11. Seaweed—Brimming with minerals, chlorophyll, and health-boosting compounds called alginates. An excellent source of natural iodine for a healthy thyroid gland.

12. Garlic—Whole baked garlic cloves help lower blood pressure and cholesterol as well as detoxifying the body from heavy metals, such as mercury and cadmium. Garlic also effectively combats many bacteria, viruses, and fungi.

PILLAR 2: EXERCISE

From head to toe, I have found that physical activity does wonders for my patients. It's absolutely essential in maintaining a healthy weight, and for individuals who are overweight or obese, diet alone cannot take and keep the weight off. Only diet and physical activity together can achieve that.

Research shows that just a minimum amount of some form of activity—a mere thirty minutes a day of walking, for instance—yields major protection, even if you are obese.

In one fascinating 2006 scientific review of the neurobiology of exercise, a group of leading researchers pointed out that regular exercise positively influences brain and nervous system function. This has "implications for the prevention and treatment of obesity, cancer, depression, the decline in cognition associated with aging, and neurological disorders such as Parkinson's disease, Alzheimer's dementia, ischemic stroke, and head and spinal cord injury," the study authors wrote, as well as reducing the effects of stress that may counteract high blood pressure, heart failure, oxidative stress, and immune deficits.

Exercise does matter, not only in the generation of growth hormone, but when it comes to improved utilization of glucose as it enters the cellular membrane. Exercise is also a great way to eliminate constipation and has been my most important recommendation for people with concerns about sluggish bowels and constipation. The elderly, who tend to be less physically active, are more vulnerable to problems of irregularity, but even light activity can make a difference. Simply walking the dog on a daily basis can be your ticket to success. Remember, healthy bowel function keeps those toxins on their way out the door!

As for myself, I walk my dogs, and ride a stationary bike or a regular bike if the weather is good. When I travel, I try to get in a workout at the hotel's fitness center.

I also work out with a personal trainer who helps me design and implement a fitness program that works for me. My overall fitness program incorporates strength training, mobility, and nutrition.

My strength training regimen includes working out with free weights twice a week. Each body part is worked once a week, with the first day focusing on chest, shoulders, and triceps. The second day we focus on legs, back, and biceps. Special workouts have been designed for the periods when I travel. Abdominals and stretching are done as part of my mobility program on both weight training days and off days, as my schedule permits.

Mobility and posture is often an area that is neglected. There are a number of factors that contribute to loss of mobility and poor posture, including injuries, aging, and spending lots of time in front of a computer screen, to name a few. A properly designed mobility program can make a world of difference.

PILLAR 3: DETOXIFICATION

We live in a toxic world. We become subtly poisoned on a daily basis, and our metabolism, enzyme systems, hormones, and vitality suffer.

The immune system—the body's guardian of health—is under constant siege, working 24/7 to destroy the impurities in the air we breathe, the food we eat, the water we drink, and the chemicals we apply to our skin.

Be mindful of the mercury found in fish, especially the deep water swimmers! Also avoid all freshwater fish. Saltwater species, such as shark, tilefish, grouper, swordfish, and large tuna, are big no-nos.

Heavy metal toxicity is one of the most significant aspects of mitochondrial poisoning. Smaller fish, such as anchovies, sardines, Boston scrod, cod, migratory Alaskan salmon, and small Atlantic halibut, are excellent choices to limit mercury exposure.

To promote your body's normal detoxification process, include high-fiber foods in your diet. Breakfast is a great meal for high-fiber cereals mixed with healthy seasonal fruits and ground flaxseed. A 25–30-gram fiber breakfast, coupled with lots of leafy-green vegetables at lunch and dinner, is a great strategy to get to 40-plus grams a day. Taking in this much fiber is a great way to enhance bowel cleansing, which will carry away toxins before they are absorbed into the body.

I also personally enjoy using a far-infrared sauna to boost my detoxification efforts. The high and dry temperatures promote vasodilation and the sweating out of toxins. Be sure to check with your doctor about using one if you have low blood pressure, are pregnant, or have any medical concerns.

Juicing is another wonderful approach to detoxification: Just follow my guidelines for selecting healthy fruits and veggies. Then juice away, whether daily or occasionally. By the way, juicing is an integral part of detoxification for those with cancer. There are plenty of great juicing recipes you can acquire when you buy a juicing machine, in books, or online (try www.drsinatra.com for some of my favorites). I also suggest the following for a simple daily detox program:

- Up to a teaspoon of vitamin C powder. Start with 1/4 teaspoon and slowly build up.

- A level teaspoon of glutamine powder. Glutamine, an amino acid, is a vital raw material for a healthy intestinal tract lining. It also helps the immune system and liver to remove toxins, including ammonia, a chemical produced from protein breakdown that contributes to neurodegenerative diseases and reduces ATP production.

- A heaping teaspoon of psyllium powder. This fibrous plant material acts like an intestinal broom, sweeping out many toxins that might otherwise be absorbed into the body.

- A daily probiotic supplement. Probiotics replenish the beneficial bacteria, such as lactobacillus, acidophilus, and bifida bacterium that reside in the intestinal tract and protect the immune system against pathogenic bacteria and candida.

PILLAR 4: MIND/BODY MEDICINE

It is no secret that optimistic people live longer than pessimistic people. When I meet patients living with catastrophic illnesses, such as heart disease, cancer, traumatic injury, and the like, I always ask about the "opportunity in crisis" as they see it.

Patients who can reframe their dilemma see their cup as half full, and often have better outcomes than those who experience their cups as half empty. If you are feeling victimized by a personal or health situation, be aware of your risk. If you lack the support or energy to turn your attitude around, seek help through family, friends, clergy, or a mental health professional.

Positive intention and a genuine belief in healing are oftentimes the most crucial aspects of dis-ease. You need to focus more on the concept that illness may be a disharmonious function in the emotional/spiritual self. Opening up to this disharmony can be the essence of gaining wisdom about the self. Remember, healing illness isn't all mechanistic. It also involves emotional and physical components which, if left unaddressed, may result in chronic, relentless disease and illness.

In order to avoid the ravages of aging, and frequently the pathological situations that accompany them, we need to focus on positive thoughts. Releasing negative thoughts, and reframing them with positive thoughts and positive intention, is a key step toward health. Remember, whatever we think becomes true, because energy follows thought. Positive intention and a positive belief in oneself are the most important aspects of staying young. To allow yourself to enjoy the simple things, such as laughing, praying, and meditating is, in itself, healing.

Meditation assuages cortisol production, the most dangerous hormone for the aging process. In addition, laughing and meditation also enhance DHEA or the "fountain of youth" hormone. Ever have an experience where you laughed so hard that you shed tears? Well, crying is the most significant release to avoid the heartbreak that often accompanies heart disease, so I encourage everyone to laugh so hard that they cry. Watch a movie that tickles your funny bone every time you see it. Relive old memories that evoke profound laughter. Keep yourself giggling by pulling a loving prank or practical joke on someone you love. Whatever it takes!

Crying also discharges blocked emotions in the body, particularly in the throat and diaphragmatic areas. Crying with sorrowful tears also releases endorphins, another anti-aging hormone, and releases tension in the throat chakra. When tears flow, surrender to them and cry it out if you can. But then forgive and forget, making the intention to move on with your life.

More than twenty years ago, I participated in an eye-opening experiment during a psychotherapy training workshop. We asked a group of forty-four male and female volunteers to discuss the most difficult issues—issues of sadness, bereavement, grief, and stress—in their lives. Afterward, we collected urine samples from them. I was amazed to find that the individuals who had talked most freely about their problems—and it was primarily women—had fewer stress breakdown chemicals in their urine, and much less evidence of cardiovascular disease. It was just the opposite for the men. We men usually have a hard time crying, or expressing emotions. This was the first time that I realized that men who don't cry or express emotion are vulnerable to cardiovascular disease.

This experiment provided the inspiration for *Heartbreak & Heart Disease*, a book I wrote in 1995, and recommend to patients because it contains lessons and stories that demonstrate how powerful a role emotions can play in healing or harming the body.

Remember to surround yourself with what you love. It may be a family, spouse, children, pets, music, plants, nature, books, or hobbies.

Whatever you love, continue to do it. I appreciate the words from Eckhart Tolle's book *The Power of Now* about staying in the present and not dwelling on the past or focusing on the future. According to Tolle—and I wholeheartedly agree—there is nothing like staying connected in the present emotion and saying yes to that moment. He chides, "What could be more futile, more insane, than to create inner resistance to something that already is? What could be more insane than to oppose life itself, which is now and always now? Surrender to what is. Say 'yes' to life—and see how life suddenly starts working for you rather than against you."

Don't forget to tell the people you love that you do love them every chance you have. I say the mantra, "love and gratitude" several times every day.

Do tai chi or yoga. Meditate. Pray. Laugh a lot. Cry. Retire later in life. Volunteer your services. Get a dog or cat that gives you unconditional love. Follow your own personal passion. Do whatever it takes to stay optimistic, happy, and engaged in life. You'll be creating the molecules of longevity.

PILLAR 5: NUTRACEUTICALS/ELECTROCEUTICALS TO ENHANCE ATP FORMATION

Electroceuticals

Electroceuticals are not the bad guys that electromagnetic fields (EMFs) are. Electromagnetic fields—or nonionizing radiation—are generated by electric power at 60 cycles AC or above. Seemingly harmless household appliances can alter cellular function, decrease levels of melatonin, and change biorhythms in a way that has a negative impact on heart-rate variability. When it comes to EMFs, you must raise your awareness about the hazards of your exposure, especially the all-too-common overuse of cellular phones and computers. The invisible waves they emit are toxic to the body. This is electropollution!

It's imperative that you limit, as much as possible, the electricity in your bedroom, where you spend one-third of your time. Watching television in bed is a problem in that regard, as are digital clocks close to the bedside. Count how many electrical devices you have in your boudoir, and start moving them. I unplug bedside lighting when I'm off to sleep, and use a grounding mattress to neutralize the electric load.

Sleeping in a grounded fashion discharges chaotic electronic exposure of the dauntless electrical sources of the day: phones, computers, cell towers, traffic, you name it! Unless you are camping out and sleeping on the ground, you may want to consider a grounding mat.

Also, avoid microwave ovens and high-tension lines. All the devices I have mentioned emit chaotic electrical cycles. It may sound insane, but I walked around my own home with an EMF detector and was appalled at the levels being emitted in the supposed safety of my own home. That's when I started rearranging furniture away from high-output outlets and made serious changes. So how do you discharge bad electromagnetic frequencies and take on healing electrons through the body? The best way is to "go grounded"; that is, go barefoot in the park, or on the beach, or in the backyard, or even on concrete for that matter. Whenever you ground the body to the earth, you not only discharge the toxic EMF in the body, you also take on healthy electrons that can combat oxidative stress. Remember that EMF frequencies can harm but, when employed consciously and correctly, they can also heal.

I wish I had the space to inform you about all the helpful electroceuticals out there. Many health care providers have programs that measure the acupuncture meridians of the body, like the Voll's. Others, like Ondamed, employ safe pulsed electromagnetic fields (PEMFs) to help their patients heal. Another positive EMF device is the far-infrared sauna.

Heat therapy was used in Spain in the 1950s to help detoxify miners from mercury poisoning. Remember, during profuse sweating, fatty tissue vibrates faster, dumping out toxins into the interstitial fluid and releasing them through the pores of the skin. Sweating eliminates toxins and also raises the pH to a more alkaline state. Sweating also is like a fever. It cooks microbes and latent viruses hidden from our immune system. A far-infrared sauna is one of the best ways to bathe the body with electromagnetic frequencies that enhance healing.

Water molecules also absorb and emit far-infrared radiation, causing water clusters to become smaller, more mobile, and easily absorbed into the tissues. Since water, particularly revitalized water, is a major component in the hydration of our cells, it is a must in the path to aging gracefully. Superior drinking water must be clean but not dead, as distilled water is.

Proper acid/base balance in the body is an important constituent in maintaining optimum health. The pH of healthy drinking water must be greater than 7.5, and the water should also be alive with photonic impulses. Cells need minerals to promote energy and enhance cellular repair. The best forms of water are revitalized waters with mineral enhancement.

Electropollution causes massive scarring of the cells, so it's absolutely essential to detoxify the body from electropollution and simultaneously maintain proper hydration. There are many vibrational waters containing homeopathic frequencies that can bring the body into proper balance. I personally purchase biological waters that you can find at www.energymedicine.org.

Supporting ATP synthesis and utilization from the nutritional and electroceutical approaches maintains the health of the cellular matrix that makes up the body. Nutraceuticals like d-ribose, the carnitines, hydrosoluble coenzyme Q_{10}, and broad-spectrum magnesium help revitalize powerful energy substrates that result in positive energy balances.

Nutraceuticals

There's no doubt about it! In our quest for optimum health, we need to take nutraceutical support in terms of a broad-spectrum, core-curriculum, nutraceutical program that includes basic vitamins and minerals and essential fatty acids. In addition to a basic foundation program with at least 1 to 2 grams of omega-3 essential fatty acids, we must also be on a mitochondrial support program that includes the awesome foursome that promotes ATP production and ATP turnover. These nutrients include:

1. Magnesium: 400–600 mg daily, especially in fractions of magnesium citrate, glycinate, taurinate, and orotate.

2. Broad-spectrum carnitine support: 500–1,500 mg doses that include L-carnitine, acetyl-L-carnitine, and propionyl L-carnitine.

3. A hydrosoluble form of coenzyme Q_{10}, usually in doses of 80–160 mg daily—more is needed for illness.

4. D-ribose: 5–10 grams daily.

This basic nutraceutical program will enhance ATP quantity and turnover, and provide nutraceutical support to mitochondria that are devoid of defense mechanisms. Mitochondrial support and membrane stabilization, taken together, are really the sine qua non of anti-aging.

In summary, the fountain of youth is right in front of us. Using strategies to optimize nutraceutical and electroceutical support improves the integrity of the cellular membrane, offering photonic impulses that enhance pulsation, increase ATP, and strengthen the vibratory activity of the cell. This is smart metabolic medicine. This is bioenergetic medicine. This is anti-aging medicine at its best.

25

Energy and Vitality

Julian Whitaker, MD

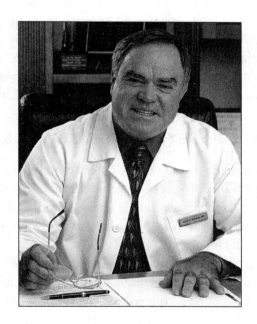

Julian Whitaker is medical director of the Whitaker Wellness Center in Newport Beach, California. He writes the *Health & Healing* newsletter and is the author of many books, including *The Whitaker Wellness Weight Loss Program*. Address: Whitaker Wellness Institute, 4321 Birch Street, Newport Beach, CA 92660. Tel: 949-851-1550. E-mail: jwhitaker @whitakerwellness.com. Website: www.whitakerwellness.com.

Health as defined by the World Health Organization is "a state of complete physical, mental, and social well-being and not just merely the absence of disease or infirmity." No argument there, but what exactly constitutes *well-being*? I think we'd all agree that one characteristic is vitality and energy. It's waking up refreshed and ready to meet the morning, and sailing through the day alert, active, and motivated.

Yet one of the most frequent complaints I hear from my patients—including those who are in pretty good health—is fatigue. They hit the snooze button a couple of times before crawling out of bed, down a few cups of coffee to get going, drag themselves through the workday, and fall asleep on the couch watching TV. Common as this scenario may be, it isn't normal, nor is it insurmountable. Although low energy could be a sign of serious disease, it's far more likely to be caused by other, often overlooked factors that, once recognized and appropriately treated, will dramatically improve your energy and quality of life.

SLEEP: BEYOND THE OBVIOUS

It's no revelation that a leading contributor to our energy crisis is poor sleep. Sleep deprivation is a serious problem that, in addition to making you feel tired, impairs mental alertness, mood, and immune function. According to research from Columbia University, skimping on sleep may even make you fat!

Conventional doctors offer vague platitudes to get more sleep, then whip out the prescription pad. Bad idea. Sleeping pills are highly addictive, and they increase the risk of cognitive problems, falls, and accidents—risks that, according to a meta-analysis published in the *British Medical Journal*, far outweigh their benefits.

Fortunately, there are a number of effective natural remedies for battling insomnia that boast impeccable safety records. My favorites include melatonin, a natural hormone that regulates the body's day-night cycles; l-theanine, an amino acid derived from green tea that increases levels of the anxiety-relieving neurotransmitter GABA; and valerian, an herbal extract touted as Europe's most popular sleep aid.

But what if you sleep eight hours a night and still drag yourself around during the day? It's possible that you are one of the 12 million

Americans who have obstructive sleep apnea, and I know from personal experience that this is a real energy zapper. Sleep apnea occurs when the fleshy tissues at the back of the throat relax and block the airway. Lack of oxygen causes the sleeper to wake briefly, gasp for breath, and then fall back to sleep. A person with severe sleep apnea may go through this routine fifteen or more times per hour. When I was tested, I had sixty-nine events in sixty minutes! This not only makes getting a good night's sleep impossible, but also dramatically increases the risk of diabetes, hypertension, stroke, heart failure, arrhythmia, and obesity.

For mild sleep apnea, weight loss, sleeping on your side, and abstaining from alcohol may be enough to prevent episodes. For moderate to severe apnea, however, the most effective treatment is a continuous positive airway pressure (CPAP) device. A mask worn over the face is attached to an air blower, which forces air through the nasal passages, keeping the airway from closing during sleep. I used to snore like a freight train until I started using a CPAP machine. Now I sleep like a baby and wake up rested and invigorated.

If you're overweight and you snore, you owe it to yourself—and your spouse and everyone else within earshot—to get tested.

LOW THYROID = LOW ENERGY

Low thyroid function as a cause of fatigue is hardly news, either. But you may be surprised by the magnitude of this problem and how often doctors miss it. Hypothyroidism affects one in thirteen Americans and as many as one in five women over age fifty. To make matters worse, more than half of them are unaware of it. This is unfortunate because besides its well-known symptoms of tiredness, weight gain, and dry skin, hypothyroidism also increases the risk of heart attack, immune dysfunction, infertility, and, to children born to women with low thyroid, neurological problems and lower IQs.

If you complain to your conventional doctor about fatigue, he'll likely test your thyroid stimulating hormone (TSH). TSH acts like a thermostat. When thyroid hormone levels are low, TSH goes up, signaling the thyroid gland to pump up production. If your TSH falls within the normal range, your doctor assumes that your thyroid is not the problem—end of story. However, you need to realize that this test is far from foolproof. It's not uncommon for someone with a normal TSH to have low levels of active thyroid hormones. At Whitaker Wellness, we treat people, not numbers. If a patient has signs and symptoms of low thyroid function, we'll offer a trial of natural thyroid replacement, regardless of test results, and such patients often respond beautifully.

Stephanie, a healthy young woman in her early thirties, came to me because she was feeling sluggish, sleeping poorly, and gaining weight. Although her TSH was normal, I placed her on a low dose of natural thyroid and asked her to monitor her body temperature when she awoke in the morning. At first, it was in the low 96s—a clear sign of hypothyroidism—but it slowly began to increase with treatment. Within months Stephanie's energy bounced back, her sleep improved, and she began getting her weight under control.

Note that I said we prescribed *natural thyroid*, not Synthroid, the most popular thyroid replacement drug on the market. The thyroid produces a number of hormones; the two most important are tri-iodothyronine (T_3) and thyroxine (T_4). Natural thyroid contains T_3, T_4, and the entire gamut of thyroid hormones, while Synthroid is a synthetic version of T_4 alone. I've never understood conventional medicine's infatuation with Synthroid. Not only is T_3 the most active thyroid hormone, but as we get older, we become less efficient at converting T_4 into T_3, which may explain the age-related rise in hypothyroidism and fatigue.

If you're chronically tired, talk to your doctor about a clinical trial of natural thyroid. If you're taking Synthroid, consider switching to natural (Armour) thyroid. If your doctor is less than helpful, look for a physician well versed in natural thyroid replacement by contacting the American College for Advancement in Medicine (ACAM; www.acamnet.org) or the American Academy of Anti-Aging Medicine (A4M; www.worldhealth.net).

BOOST YOUR ENERGY WITH TARGETED NUTRIENTS

I'm often asked about products that claim to increase energy. Do they work? Without a doubt, caffeine (the "active" ingredient in Red Bull and other energy drinks and supplements) gives you a jolt of energy. It's a central nervous system stimulant that triggers the fight-or-flight response and thus increases mental alertness and physical perform-ance. I personally start my mornings with a cup or two of coffee and, given caffeine's diverse health benefits, I give moderate consumption a thumbs-up.

However, when patients ask for help with persistent fatigue, I don't send them to Starbucks. Instead, I recommend that they head to the health food store to pick up a potent daily multivitamin and mineral supplement. Surveys reveal that Americans are woefully deficient in a number of vitamins and minerals involved in energy production. For example, 56 percent of us don't get enough magnesium, and up to 20 percent of women have anemia due to iron deficiency. Low levels of vitamin B_{12} are also common, especially as we get older, and supple-mental B_{12} can work wonders in restoring flagging energy.

Once the basic vitamin and mineral requirements are covered, I focus on supporting the mitochondria. Adenosine triphosphate (ATP), the energy that fuels the cells, is synthesized entirely within the mito-chondria, and, as you can imagine, keeping up with the body's enor-mous energy demands is no easy task. Furthermore, generating ATP is risky business for the mitochondria because highly damaging free radicals are an inevitable by-product of the process. Oxidative dam-age takes its toll, and over the years mitochondria become less effi-cient, resulting in an energy slowdown that underlies the entire aging process.

To keep your cellular power plants in peak condition, start by tak-ing coenzyme Q_{10}. CoQ_{10} is sometimes referred to as the spark plug of the energy-producing system, and relatively small CoQ_{10} deficien-cies can have significant effects on cellular energy. In addition to ensuring sufficient energy production, supplemental CoQ_{10} is a potent antioxidant that protects against free radical damage. Another important antioxidant is alpha-lipoic acid (ALA). Unlike other free radical scavengers, ALA is both water-soluble and fat-soluble, mean-ing it provides protection in all parts of the cell, and it is particularly active in the mitochondria.

The final energy-boosting supplement I want to tell you about is ribose, a simple, five-carbon sugar that serves as the structural backbone of ATP. Simply put, if your cells don't have enough ribose, they'll run out of juice. When taken orally, ribose is delivered to energy-starved tissues, where it rapidly and dramatically rebuilds energy reserves. This supplement is particularly effective in restoring energy to the heart muscle, and studies show that it increases activity levels in patients with heart failure and coronary artery disease. It's also an excellent therapy for fibromyalgia and chronic fatigue, and athletes take it to speed recovery and improve endurance.

THE BLESSING OF ABUNDANT ENERGY

I would be remiss if I didn't mention the importance of lifestyle changes for restoring energy. First, you need to exercise. I know what you're thinking—when you're pooped, the last thing you want to do is exercise, but inactivity nurtures a vicious cycle of even more fatigue that can only be broken by physical activity. In a 2008 study, researchers from the University of Georgia discovered that when tired, unmotivated couch potatoes engaged in a program of low-intensity exercise, their fatigue decreased by 65 percent and their energy levels increased by 20 percent.

Second, evaluate your diet. If you have tired spells that come on in the midmorning or midafternoon, you may be suffering from low blood sugar. Rather than eating three large meals a day, break them into five smaller meals or snacks, and make sure each includes a moderate amount of protein. Eliminate starches and sugars entirely. These quick-burning carbohydrates cause extreme highs and lows in blood sugar, which can result in decreased energy, difficulty concentrating, and food cravings.

If you feel the need to get a little vim and vigor back into your life, make sure you're getting enough sleep, check your thyroid function, take targeted supplements, exercise regularly, and clean up your diet. After all, abundant energy is the essence of health.

Afterword

As the editor of *The Fountain*, I was fascinated by the personal experiences ad recommendations of our experts. Many of them became advocates of nutritional therapies after successfully using diet and nutritional supplements to resolve their own health problems. One important lesson I drew from the essays is that no single nutrition or lifestyle plan fits everyone. Given our genetic and biochemical individuality (or diversity, if you prefer), *your* path to a long and healthy life may be a little like shopping for clothes: "Try on" different ideas and concepts to see what "fits you best." How will you know you're on the right track? Having good, steady energy levels (without taking a lot of stimulants) and a sense of well-being are good indicators of overall health.

I found it interesting that extreme calorie restriction, one of the best-researched aspects of anti-aging medicine, was noted only briefly. Calorie restriction extends life span by slowing down metabolic processes, and it was first shown to slow the aging process in rodents in the 1930s. In small-mammal studies, cutting calorie consumption by about 30 percent early in life led to a 30 percent increase in life expectancy. Primate studies involving calorie restriction have been underway for many years, and so far they also point to a lower risk of age-related diseases, such as diabetes, cancer, and heart disease— which would be consistent with increased life expectancy.

Extreme calorie-restricted diets do have serious practical drawbacks, and only a few brave souls have adopted them. People on such diets have told me that they have lost weight, but to the point of being emaciated, and they are almost always hungry and cold. Although people might want to live longer, most would probably like an easier, less extreme way of doing so. An easier way may emerge in the next few years. For example, animal studies have found that supplemental chromium and resveratrol result in cellular changes similar to those that occur on low-calorie diets.

EATING HABITS

The late nutrition educator Carlton Fredericks, PhD, observed that nutrition experts have recommended a wide variety of diets and foods for health, but that there is only one food we know we were meant to consume: breast milk during infancy.

Beyond that, what might people eat to maintain their health and live a healthy and long life? Loren Cordain, PhD, looked to the past for our dietary baseline, focusing on the types of foods our genes codeveloped with over long spans of time. During these many years of human development, people subsisted primarily on two food groups: (1) lean animal proteins and fish, and (2) vegetables and fruits. Grains (whole and refined), legumes, dairy, processed oils, and refined sugars did not become part of human diets until relatively recently, genetically speaking. As a result, most foods other than lean proteins and produce are a genetic mismatch for us, increasing the risk of disease. Based on Cordain's data, and that of anthropological studies of pretechnological cultures, a traditional diet that focuses on protein and produce appears to protect against chronic degenerative diseases.

A modern version of the Paleolithic (or Stone Age) diet is actually very simple to follow. It does require cooking food largely from scratch, but the time involved in grocery shopping is significantly reduced. A modern Paleolithic-style diet would be built around fish, fowl, eggs, lean meats, and ample amounts of high-fiber (nonstarchy) vegetables and fruits. People who exercise regularly could certainly consume a little more starch. Other food products, such as bread, legumes, and cheese, would best be treated as occasional treats rather than staples.

Contributors who discussed nutrition were in agreement on what to avoid, particularly refined foods, trans fats, and large amounts of omega-6 fats (found in most cooking oils). Indeed, half of any sound nutrition program in the twenty-first century would have to avoid most of the artifacts of modern, processed, denatured foods. When you eliminate all or nearly all processed junk foods, what you have left are fresh foods. At that point, it almost does not matter whether you opt for an omnivore diet, a vegetarian diet, a Japanese diet, or a Mediterranean diet, because you have eliminated nutritionally empty or negative foods. (I use the term *negative* to reflect how some unhealthy foods, such as sugars and refined carbohydrates, actually reduce the body's levels of vitamin B_1 and chromium.)

Food Allergies

Even the healthiest foods can be unhealthy if you happen to be allergic to them. James Braly, MD, an expert on food and chemical sensitivities, addressed the confounding nature of food allergies. Food allergies can be considered the "great mimicker" because they can cause or exacerbate symptoms of most other diseases, including arthritis and mood disorders. Too often, food allergies are overlooked in conventional medicine.

Do you have food allergies? One of the classic methods of identifying them is to consider the foods you crave or can't imagine living without. The reason is that people are often addicted to the very foods they are allergic to. Although this allergy-addiction pattern might seem strange, it is supported by decades of clinical and research experience. As Dr. Braly explains, more sophisticated testing can confirm the presence of food allergies.

The best and simplest way to identify and correct food allergies is through avoidance of the suspect food. The most common food allergens are wheat, dairy, corn, and soy. The first few days of avoidance can be difficult because of the addiction aspect. Avoidance also demands that people carefully read food labels, or ask specific questions about ingredients (such as flour as a sauce thickener) in restaurants. Sometimes, after several months or years, you can regain some degree of tolerance for the problematic foods. However, you must be careful to avoid consuming the food on a regular basis or risk it becoming an allergen again.

NUTRITIONAL SUPPLEMENTS

If the Paleolithic diet forms our genetic or biological baseline for nutrition, orthomolecular nutrition sets the goal for optimizing our nutrient intake. The term *orthomolecular* essentially means using nutrients to create an optimal molecular environment within our bodies Our entire biochemistry, including the activities of our genes, depends on nutrients. Each of us inherits or develops biochemical weaknesses, and the selective use of supplements can often correct for these weaknesses. Ideally, it would be best to have a nutritionally oriented physician measure our nutrient levels; doing so takes the guesswork out of deciding which supplements to take. In fact, many nutritionally oriented physicians do such measurements. However, most people don't opt for such nutrient assessments, and you can follow some general guidelines.

First, nutritional deficiencies (or borderline "insufficiencies") are frightfully common in the United States. So a reasonable starting assumption is that you are either deficient or have a marginal intake of at least one nutrient. Many factors, including drugs (such as acid-blockers and oral contraceptives), interfere with the absorption or utilization of nutrients, further compromising the nutritional health of millions of people. Because of widespread nutritional deficiencies, and because the official governmental recommendations are too low for optimal health, it is important to take a high-potency multivitamin plus a multimineral supplement. Treat these multis as the foundation of your nutritional supplement program.

Second, give serious thought to building on these multis with individual supplements tailored to your individual nutritional, biochemical, and genetic requirements. To do this, look at your own health and patterns of disease in your family, and read as much as you can about nutrition and health. (After all, you are your own best second opinion.) For example, if you are at increased risk of diabetes, you may want to take extra chromium, biotin, alpha-lipoic acid, or silymarin. If you are at increased risk of heart failure or cancer, consider taking extra coenzyme Q_{10} and L-carnitine, which are vitaminlike nutrients.

Third, our bodies do deteriorate with age, our nutrient reserves tend to decrease, and our biochemistry becomes less efficient. We can offset or slow down many of these changes by selectively "loading" our biochemical pathways with higher amounts of nutrients. For example, coenzyme Q_{10} plays essential roles in the conversion of food to energy, and it also limits the release of harmful by-products from this normal metabolic process. One of the traits of aging is a decline in energy, and coenzyme Q_{10} can compensate for some of that. Another trait of aging is frailty related to weak muscles and bones. In this case, vitamin D can help maintain normal muscle and bone.

PHYSICAL ACTIVITY

Physical activity is also essential for maintaining health, and the greater your daily physical activity, the healthier you will likely be. Physical activity can include walking, gardening, housecleaning, and dancing. In fact, simply going for a brisk daily walk for thirty to forty minutes can significantly lower blood sugar and insulin levels, lowering the risk of diabetes and heart disease. A structured exercise program, including running, swimming, or bicycling, may yield even greater benefits.

Unfortunately, many people don't exercise because they either "don't have the time" or because they are too tired. The first couple of weeks or so of an exercise program may, in fact, leave you feeling more tired. This is a result of muscle fatigue, and it will start to resolve as you strengthen your muscles. All of us can make time for physical activity, such as going for a walk during lunch, if we choose to do so. If you feel that your life is too busy or hectic to include regular physical activity or exercise, it may be a sign that you have to reset your priorities for health and longevity.

REDUCING STRESS

A little bit of stress can increase creativity and productivity. Too much stress, however, leads to elevated and sustained levels of cortisol, a destructive stress hormone. High levels of cortisol are strongly associated with unhealthy aging and a greater risk of disease.

It's nearly impossible to avoid stress in our world, so the key is to manage it and reduce its negative impact on our health. There are many ways to do this. Breathing exercises, including just three or four slow deep breaths, can quickly reduce stress levels. Downtime, such as reading, hobbies, and vacations can also reduce stress. Yoga and meditation are well known for their stress-buffering benefits. However, if your life is particularly stressful, it is important to build regular stress-reducing activities into your daily schedule and not wait to take an annual vacation.

Some of us actually increase our stress as a way of getting an adrenalin rush—that is, we seek out stress rather than avoiding it. One of the most common ways we do this is by being emotionally reactive to stressful situations. We might respond angrily to work pressures, another driver, or a comment from a spouse. Being reactive tends to escalate the situation and the stress, along with elevating cortisol levels and blood pressure. Although it takes a little self-training not to be reactive (and instead to remain somewhat emotionally detached), it does blunt the effects of many stresses.

EMOTIONAL HEALTH AND RELATIONSHIPS

In his chapter, Ron Hunninghake, MD, succinctly forged the link between emotions and health with an example many of us have unfortunately uttered at least once: "I'm sick and tired of you." Unhealthy relationships set the stage for sickness, whereas healthy relationships set the stage for good health! Nearly all the conflicts we wrestle with in life are the result of unresolved relationship issues.

According to Hunninghake, the biggest danger to healthy relationships is wanting to control another person. This type of control is more common and often more subtle than you might think. If some people frustrate you or make you angry, it is almost always because they are not doing what you would like them to do. If you try to control that person's actions, your desire to control will inevitably conflict with the other person's need for freedom. People often try to control another person by criticizing, blaming, complaining, nagging, threatening, punishing, or bribing.

"Healthy relationships," Hunninghake writes, "are built on the assumption of the intrinsic freedom of choice"—that is, the decision to be in a relationship. He cites seven ingredients (originally developed by Dr. William Glasser) in healthy relationships: listening, supporting, encouraging, respecting, trusting, accepting, and always negotiating disagreements.

FAITH

Faith can take many different forms, and it contributes to longevity. Studies have found that religious individuals tend to live longer than those who are less religious, though there are likely other variables, such as a stronger family and social network among more devout individuals.

Faith can be expressed through religion or more general feelings of "belief." Many people describe themselves as spiritual but not religious; they may believe in God, but dislike organized religion. And there are many variations on the theme of faith, spirituality, and religiosity. I know an atheist who is extraordinarily spiritual. He sees his place in the universe in the context of biological evolution.

STRIVE FOR BALANCE

It is easy to become obsessed with nutrition or exercise—or any other single aspect of health—but achieving a balance in your life activities is crucial to longevity. An example: Workaholics aren't fun to hang around with. Their lives are unbalanced, and they tend to rationalize their behavior and long hours with a lot of "have tos."

It's rare to achieve balance every single day (and attempting to do so may be a sign of overstructuring your life), but such balance can be maintained on a weekly basis. I'll offer myself as an example. At one time, I would have been considered a workaholic, working six and a half days a week, including many evenings. My typical week is still filled with a variety of deadlines for different magazines, newsletters, and publishers. However, I now end most of my workdays between five and six o'clock—that's a personal boundary so work does not disrupt the rest of my life. Some of my balance comes from bicycling three to four mornings a week, which provides both a time for exercise and a rhythm that encourages meditationlike reflection and emotional processing. Cooking also is often a meditationlike experience for me: I enjoy the tactile nature of cutting up food and the creativity of making a meal. Fine-art photography is another counterbalance to my deadlines. To explain, writing for magazines and books is usually a collaborative effort, with editors routinely asking questions and requesting changes. My "ownership" of my writing is limited under these circumstances. By contrast, I am able to maintain complete creative control of my photography, requiring me to satisfy no one but myself. Think of balance as musical counterpoint—two different themes that merge together nicely.

The lesson? Nutrition, supplements, and physical activity are cornerstones for health and longevity. But never neglect the creative, emotional, and spiritual aspects of health. You will always be an individual, and you will always be part of a network of family, friends, and life. ***Live long!***

Index